Therapy Outcome Measure
User Guide and Scales

Therapy Outcome Measure
User Guide and Scales

Pam Enderby and Alexandra John

J&R Press Ltd

Library of Congress Cataloguing in Publication Data
British Library Cataloguing in Publication Data
A catalogue record for this book is available from the British Library
Cover design: Jim Wilkie. Cover image: Clive Watts/Shutterstock.
Project management, typesetting and design: J&R Publishing Services Ltd, Guildford,
Surrey, UK; www.jr-publishingservices.co.uk
Printed and bound by CPI Group (UK) Ltd, Croydon, CR0 4YY

To access the downloads that accompany this book use the following URL:
www.jr-press.co.uk/therapy-outcome-download.zip

Contents

"The ultimate goal is to manage quality, but you cannot manage it until you have a way to measure it, and you cannot measure it until you can monitor it."

Florence Nightingale

Foreword

Outcome measurement is essential for demonstrating the delivery of high quality and effective services, as well as examining the impact of interventions. The Therapy Outcome Measures for Rehabilitation Professionals (TOM) (Enderby & John, 1997; Enderby, John, & Petheram, 2006; Enderby & John, 2015) was designed to be a simple, reliable, cross-disciplinary and cross-client group method of gathering information on a broad spectrum of issues associated with therapy/rehabilitation. The TOM assists services to review their strengths and weaknesses. Its validity and reliability have been established (Bowen et al., 2012; Enderby et al., 2012; Enderby & John, 2015; Hammerton, 2004; Hesketh et al., 2011; John, 2001; Palmer et al., 2018; Roulstone et al., 2004; Ryan, 2003). It is an approach which enables allied health professionals (AHPs), nurses, and other health, education and social care professionals to describe the relative abilities of an individual across four dimensions, which cover both health and social aspects, at the beginning, during and at the end of an intervention.

One of the essential requirements of any outcome measure, whether subjective or objective, is to ensure that the results are reliable and reflect the situation appropriately. This requires more consideration than looking at a scale and attributing a number that seems right! It is important that the philosophy, structure and terminology are understood as well as the process. Thus, before using any measure, including the TOM, you will need to consider the essential ingredients which are outlined in this user guide.

The dimensions are based on those described by the World Health Organisation's International Classification of Disability and Function (WHO, ICF, 2001):

1. Impairment: the underlying condition
2. Activity: ability to complete daily activities
3. Participation: social participation
4. Wellbeing: emotional health. This domain is not included in the WHO ICF 2001 but was added to the TOM as goals of health and rehabilitation services were frequently related to improving wellbeing.

> "The ICF is a scientific tool for consistent, internationally comparable information about the experience of health and disability. As such, it also provides the basis for WHO overall approach to health."
> *http://www.who.int/classifications/icf/icfbeginnersguide.pdf*

The TOM can be used with a range of different client groups, either as a unidisciplinary or a multidisciplinary rating tool.

This user guide will assist practitioners to:

- Understand the purposes and underlying principles of the Therapy Outcome Measure (TOM)
- Comprehend the principles
- Use the approach reliably
- Implement the TOM in your service
- Conduct a basic analysis of the data you have collected.

The authors, Pam Enderby and Alex John, appreciate the considerable assistance provided by Kathryn Moyse in the preparation of this User Guide. Her practical approach and attention to detail has been invaluable.

For more detailed information relating to the development and psychometrics please see: Enderby P. & John A. (2015). *Therapy Outcome Measures for Rehabilitation Professionals*, 3rd edition. Guildford: J&R Press.

Contact details:
Pam Enderby p.m.enderby@sheffield.ac.uk
Alex John speechandlanguage.ajohn@gmail.com

1 Understanding the basics

This chapter provides a step-by-step guide for getting familiar with the TOM. For further information about the domains of the TOM, please refer to Chapters 2 and 3.

Step 1 Understanding the domains of the TOM

It is essential that a user of the measure has a good understanding of the different domains and the issues to be considered when making a judgement. The definitions are based on those developed by the WHO ICF (excepting wellbeing).

Impairment

Impairment is concerned with the integrity of body systems, and includes psychological and physiological structures. It reflects the disease or medical disorder experienced by the individual. The medical diagnosis is embraced in this domain.

Impairments include: stroke, learning disability, autism, diabetes, musculoskeletal conditions, respiratory disorders, schizophrenia, dysphagia, language disorder, etc.

Activity/disability/functioning

These terms are all concerned with what someone can do and these terms are frequently used interchangeably. They describe the ability to execute tasks and/or limitations on actions by an individual, indicating the level of dependence and independence. This domain concerns the degree of abnormality (as compared to someone of the same age, gender and culture) in terms of difference from the norm of what someone undertakes.

Activities include: walking, communicating, reading, washing, etc.

Participation

Participation is concerned with the advantage/disadvantage experienced by the individual, reflecting social participation, integration, interaction, and autonomy. It reviews the individual in a social setting and reflects access to the environment, employment, recreation, education and family participation.

Participation includes: having hobbies, friends, autonomy, getting out, being respected, etc.

Wellbeing/distress

This domain is concerned with emotions, feelings, burden of upset, concern and anxiety, and level of satisfaction. This domain is not included in the WHO ICF 2001 but was added to the first edition of the *Therapy Outcome Measure* (Enderby, John, & Petheram, 1999) following a review of goals of therapists and rehabilitation services where it was found that improving the wellbeing of the individual as well as their family members or carers was a frequent goal/objective of services and therefore needed to be included in the review of outcomes of those services.

There are two concepts related to wellbeing: the first is related to the **severity** of any upset, concern, anxiety, anger (how severe), and the second is related to the **frequency** of experiencing this, e.g., all the time, frequently, often. So, for example, one should consider whether the person is extremely anxious/depressed all of the time, or occasionally gets very cross, or frequently gets mildly cross, and so on.

Carer wellbeing scale

If one of the objectives of the intervention is to improve the wellbeing of the carer of the client, then it may be appropriate to reflect this by using the same wellbeing scale to determine the level of challenge experienced by the carer at the beginning and the end of the intervention. In some cases this may be the only objective of an intervention.

Do not use this scale if the management of this is not part of your intervention plan or you do not see/know the carers.

Step 2 Explaining the rating scale

The TOM domains (impairment, activity, participation, and wellbeing) are rated on an **ordinal** rating scale*, with 0 representing the severe end of the scale and 5 being considered normal for the age, sex, and culture of the client.

0	0.5	1	2	2.5	3	3.5	4	4.5	5

The integers (whole numbers) are given a description that identifies the severity of the difficulty experienced on each dimension. Half points increase the scale to 11 points. The half points (which have no descriptor) allow the assessor to indicate whether the person is better or worse than what is described. In summary, there are six descriptions on each scale and five undefined half points providing an 11-point scale (see Step 4 below).

When using the scales, the assessor should identify the point on the scale that is 'best fit'; it is not essential that the individual presents with all of the features described. The half points on the scale can assist with this. For example, if the individual presents with some of the features described in the descriptor for '4' and some in '3', it may be appropriate to score a 3.5.

---

*A **scale** on which data is shown simply in order of magnitude since there is no standard of measurement of differences: it is possible to order the variables by ranking them with the differences between scale points varying in size and so reflect that one person is better than another, but not by how much.

What does a change of 0.5 mean?

A clinically significant change is defined as 'the practical importance of a treatment effect – where it has a real genuine, palpable, noticeable effect on daily life'. Indeed, defining meaningful change, in terms of either improvement or worsening (aggravation), is a complicated issue and involves clinical, personal, and statistical considerations. However, change relates very intimately to the concept of difference and is judged based on and relating to a time span, that is, the smallest difference in the domain of interest which is perceived as beneficial or important between two time points (Rai, Yazdany, Fortin, & Aviña-Zubieta, 2015). It therefore represents a threshold for outcome scores (either patient-reported or clinician-measured) over which either would consider a given change in score to be meaningful and worthwhile.

"Change invariably relates to a difference in some measurable entity and almost always it relates to a time span. The confirmation of clinical change is important both for varying the treatment course (if necessary) and for the termination of treatment when the latter has reached either its prescribed objective or a plateau. Since in the context of rehabilitation, the outcome measures (OM) are strongly linked to performance, determination of change in the latter is confounded by many factors, collectively known as the error of measurement, which render a decision regarding clinically meaningful change, highly involved."
(Dvir, 2015)

For the TOM, this is set at 0.5. (Further information on using 0.5 when rating, please see **Arm's-length change** (page 10)).

Step 3 When to rate

All outcome measures endeavour to examine change associated with a course of action or treatment. Thus, the TOM is used at the beginning and the end of an intervention. This can be one session if that session was an intervention that effected change.

Admission/start rating

The procedures for using the TOM requires you as the health/education/social care professional to assess the individual referred for treatment using your usual assessment procedures, such as standardized tests, observation, reports from others, and consideration of medical and social history. Thus, no additional work/assessments or tests are required.

A rating should be ascribed to an individual when you are ready to start your treatment/intervention but of course it is important that you have all relevant information beforehand. With some individuals, you will be able to do this fairly quickly having received the referral, taken a case history, interviewed and observed. With other clients you will need to get more information which may take several weeks as you will need to undertake a range of assessments, and discuss with relevant others such as teachers, other health professionals or family members. It is only after you have gathered this information that you will be able to decide on a treatment approach or intervention programme for that episode of care. So in this case it would be at this point that you would rate the individual. The information gained can then be organized into the four dimensions of the TOM so the behaviours can be described ready to rate using the descriptors.

Intermediate ratings

Ratings can be made at any point in the episode of care to assess what has changed or been maintained. It is sometimes necessary to do an intermediate rating in order to monitor progress, discuss at a case conference, or support a report. Intermediate ratings may be useful at certain points and there is no limit to the numbers of these that you can do.

Final/discharge rating

At the end of an episode of care a final rating should be made. This may or may not be the end of care for that individual; you may wish to change the treatment plan, emphasizing a new area for intervention.

End of episode/discharge codes can be used to indicate whether the individual has been discharged from the service or will continue to receive treatment.

Explaining an episode of care

An episode of care is a period of treatment or intervention with a defined aim or aims. There may be several episodes of care in the management of an individual. Each episode of care may require a different TOM scale to be used (see Step 4, below). It is important that the same scale is used when rating the individual at the beginning of the episode of care and the end of the episode of care, to enable change to be measured (see Figure 1.1).

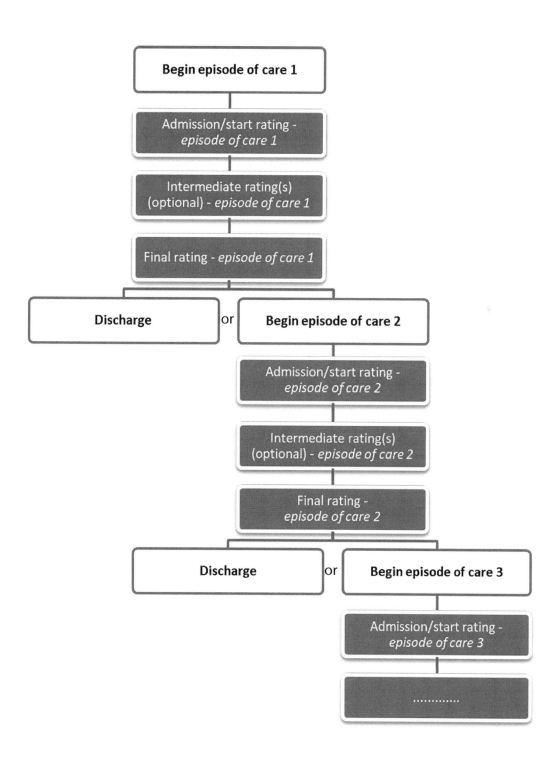

Figure 1.1 An episode of care.

Table 1.1 An example of a final/discharge rating.

End of episode/discharge code	Definition	Episode of care completed?
End of episode of care (to be reviewed)	The goals of treatment for the episode of care are complete. Further intervention required.	Yes
Therapy complete (discharged)	SLT is complete and there is no need for further SLT at this time	Yes
Transferred to another service	Individual was transferred to another service before completing the episode of care	No
Did not attend	Episode of care terminated because the individual did not attend	No
Died	Individual died during the episode of care	Yes/no
Moved out of area	Individual moved out of area before completing the episode of care	No
Intervening illness	Individual experiences an illness during the episode of care which affects the goals of treatment	No
Different intervention required	During the course of the episode of care, the goals of treatment were changed	No
Unknown/other	The reason for the end of the episode of care is not specified or not known	Not known

The following case studies provide examples of episodes of care.

Bert, aged 4, has a phonological problem and is hyperactive

Episode of care 1

Objective: To reduce the hyper-anxiety of mother related to Bert's speech and her tendency to overcorrect.

SLT explains Bert's difficulty with discriminating between sounds and the importance of encouraging listening. Models the methods of engaging and rewarding Bert.

3 sessions

Episode of care 2

Objective: To improve auditory attention. SLT engages Bert with games, rewarding discrimination between dissimilar sounds. Additional reward for increasing length of time engaged on game.

4 sessions

Episode of care 3

Bert is entering school and has become anxious that he is not being understood by new classmates.

Objective: To improve articulation accuracy and communication skills.

SLT explains new objectives to mother – encourage Bert to use gesture and undertake sound practice in games at home. Emphasize rewarding when communicating clearly.

5 sessions

Margaret, aged 82, has had a stroke

Episode of care 1

Objective: To improve symmetry in walking.

Episode of care 2

Objective: To increase confidence in walking.

Episode of care 3

Objective: To include carers with Margaret to develop a self-management plan aimed at prevention of falls.

Peter, aged 18, has a severe hidden stammer

Episode of care 1

Objective: Reducing anxiety associated with speaking by improving understanding of fluency disorder and exploring Peter's reactions and insight. Encouragement to discuss fluency disorder with friends.
4 sessions

Episode of care 2

Objective: Encouragement of more expressive/overt dysfluency.
3 sessions

Episode of care 3

Management strategies for dysfluency without word avoidance. Assignments given for practice and to increase social participation.
3 sessions

Step 4 Choosing a scale

Once you have gathered sufficient information about the individual to identify the focus of the intervention, it is then appropriate to identify which TOM scale to use.

The core scale

The core scale has an operationally-defined severity scale from profound to normal with limited descriptions detailing the core concepts of impairment, activity, participation and wellbeing. This can be used for clients where an adapted scale is not available or is inappropriate. See details of the core scale on page 54.

Table 1.2 TOM ordinal scale.

Profound		Severe		Severe/ Moderate		Moderate		Mild		Normal
0	0.5	1	1.5	2	2.5	3	3.5	4	4.5	5

Adapted scales

A number of more detailed 'adapted' scales (>50) have been developed to facilitate rating on the TOM by providing expanded descriptions for different client groups. These assist with improving agreement between raters (interrater reliability) which can be difficult when such terms as 'moderate' are interpreted differently by different raters. The adapted scales have been developed by experts working with the specified client groups and have been tested for their reliability (unless otherwise stated).

These scales broadly follow the same structure as the core scale, requiring the assessor to rate the individual on the domains of impairment, activity, participation and wellbeing using detailed descriptors. Some scales, such as the AAC scale, have a slightly different structure. The adapted scales can be found on page 47.

Accompanying scales

Some services have developed additional scales which assist them to extend the use of TOM by collecting additional information related to the objectives of an episode of care in a consistent manner (see page 259).

Choosing the right scale

Use the adapted scale most appropriate for the client and the focus of intervention for the current care episode. You may find that a number of the scales would be appropriate to use with the individual.

Note the scale used so that when the case is reviewed it is rated on the same scale.

Using more than one scale

If the individual has more than one condition that you are working on, you can rate them on more than one scale. It is recommended that the primary condition for the referral to your service is used first. For example, an individual who has a learning difficulty is referred because of a musculoskeletal problem. You would rate using the musculoskeletal adapted scale first and the learning disability scale second.

Whilst it is reasonably easy to discriminate the impact/severity of two impairments, it may be more difficult to discriminate between which of these is having the greater impact on two 'activities' in some cases. Therefore, you could rate two impairments separately but only rate one 'activity' domain unless these are clearly distinct as in the example of 'activity' for dysphasia (communication) and 'activity' for dysphagia (swallowing).

Generally, you should only rate 'participation' and 'wellbeing' once as it has been found to be difficult to distinguish the impact of more than one condition on these domains. Thus, you can rate up to two impairments, up to two activities, but rate a singular participation and wellbeing.

If the individual has three conditions, for example has had a stroke, has a mental health condition and cognitive disorder, you should use either the Multifactorial Conditions or the Complex and Multiple Difficulties adapted scales as it has been found to be difficult to discriminate the impact of each condition and how they individually influence and add a degree of complexity to the rehabilitation process.

Changing the scale midway through therapy

Occasionally, you will begin therapy with an individual on the basis of a particular diagnosis only to find at a later stage that that individual has a different diagnosis. Alternatively, there may be an intervening illness, and/or the priority for that individual may have changed meaning that a different intervention is required. You may have rated the individual on a particular adapted scale and undertaken an intervention based upon that information, but subsequently you need to change the approach to the therapy as the new information changes your understanding of the underlying impairment. In these situations, it is recommended that you do a final/discharge rating (using the same scale as you used previously) and use the discharge/end of episode of care code 'different intervention required' or 'intervening illness' or another appropriate code, then proceed as with a new patient using a new admission/start rating on the appropriate scale.

How do I rate a patient/client with varying ability?

Capability versus performance

One of the objectives of therapy may be to reduce variation. It is always encouraging when you find that the client can occasionally do something well as it indicates that this level is within their repertoire and you will want to reduce the variation and increase the performance to be consistently at the best level possible. Furthermore, it has been found that when making a subjective judgement it is easier to achieve consistency if you rate more harshly than more generously. Thus, you should rate on the most consistent lower end of the individual's behaviour/presentation.

Arm's-length change

Every therapist has techniques which are often nonverbal and can indicate encouragement to the patient. These may lead to the individual performing at a higher level than they usually do when relaxed and in their own environment. You should attempt to rate behaviours that can be seen by others, and when observing the behaviours ask yourself: "Would this be evident to another person?"

How long does it take to rate a client?

The TOM takes a short time to administer, as ratings are only allocated when the individual has been assessed or reassessed and goals set. Whilst it will often take up to 10 minutes when you start to use TOM, it will only take 2-3 minutes (including completing documentation) once you have become familiar with the approach.

A useful approach is to think of whether the individual is likely to be at the top end, bottom end or middle of a particular domain scale. That is, would the behaviours be ranked 'mild', 'moderate' or 'severe'? Then you will only need to read and consider 2 scale points.

Step 5 Get familiar with ICD codes

In addition to recording which scale you use, it can be useful to record additional diagnostic information about the individual you are working with. Standardized coding systems can assist with recording this information in a consistent and systematic manner. The World Health Organisation has developed the International Classification of Diseases and Related Health Problems (ICD) to assist with this.

You may wish to code:

- the medical diagnosis
- any relevant underlying difficulties.

Doing this helps you to understand the complexity of the condition(s) and other factors that may influence the outcomes, and will be useful when it comes to analyzing the data you have collected (see Chapter 4). For example, if you are working on developing the expressive language skills of a young child with a learning disability, it may be helpful to record this information using ICD codes in addition to the TOM scale you have chosen (Language Disorder/Developmental Language Disorder). It would be appropriate to analyze the outcomes of these children and compare the results with children with Developmental Language Disorder, in which the language difficulties are not associated with an underlying biomedical condition. Another example is if you are working with an individual with a hip replacement who has a neurological disorder; it may be helpful to record this information (Parkinson's Disease) using the ICD codes in addition to the TOM scale you have chosen. To find relevant ICD10 code go to http://apps.who.int/classifications/icd10/browse/2016/en and use the search function.

Collecting this information can also be useful where there is no adapted scale for the condition you are focusing on and you use the core scale.

You may wish to devise a 'shortlist' of codes to use in your department for ease of use and to ensure consistency.

References

Dvir, Z. (2015). Difference, significant difference and clinically meaningful difference: The meaning of change in rehabilitation. *Journal of Exercise Rehabilitation*, *11*(2), 67-73. doi:10.12965/jer.150199

Rai, S.K., Yazdany, J., Fortin, P.R., & Aviña-Zubieta, J.A. (2015). Approaches for estimating minimal clinically important differences in systemic lupus erythematosus. *Arthritis Research Therapy*, *17*, 143. doi: 10.1186/s13075-015-0658-6

2 Introducing the TOM to your service

Prior to using TOM it is useful to become familiar with the approach and to practise rating. You may wish to do this with your colleagues. Discussion can help to clarify certain principles of its usage and ensure that each staff member has a good understanding of the philosophical underpinning and practical issues in its application. The group discussion may be assisted by the following format:

- Discussion regarding need for outcome measurement.
- Discussion regarding dimensions of impairment, activity restriction, social participation and wellbeing (of both patients and carer). Discuss the ICF and its principles – it is essential for all staff members to have a clear understanding of the difference between the domains.
- Practise rating patients/clients/students (see following text for suggestions).
- Practise completing data collection forms and coding.
- Come to an agreement on:
  - pilot/trial study period.
  - who to score (which patient/client group – all or particular ones)?
  - when you will begin using the TOM – with just new referrals or individuals already on the caseload?
  - are you using the TOM as a uni-professional tool or as an integrated team?
  - how and where will you record the information?
  - who analyzes the data/understands how to analyze data?
  - who/how to train new staff members, locums and staff on rotation (please ensure that the induction programme for new members of staff includes basic information and details regarding TOM).
  - when and how to review outcome reports.

It is essential for the success of any outcome initiative, whether using this measure or another, to have a clearly defined and agreed action plan that reflects the new activity.

Practising using the TOM

The first training session should allow the therapists to gain a clear understanding of the underlying purpose, principles and structures of the TOM.

1. Use case studies to identify which aetiology is present and the aims and objectives of the episode of intervention.

2. Practise selecting the correct ICD code.

3. Decide which features of a case history or any assessments you undertake would assist you in rating the different dimensions of impairment, activity, participation and wellbeing.

4. Use the core scale or the appropriate adapted scale to reflect your clinical judgement.

5. Remind yourself and the group that the client does not have to have every feature as specified in the scale; consider which description best fits the presentation of the client.

6. Group practice in the use of the tool to achieve consistency in rating is valuable. For example, you could ask each member of the group to describe one of their own cases (see suggested method of presentation below). The group members first rate that case independently and then as a group. The discussion on rating each dimension helps to establish consistency and stability in rating on the TOM. After rating 10 cases, the speed of completing a rating, as well as the reliability, increases.

7. Identify how to implement use of the TOM in a clinical setting.

8. Agree on an action plan and dates for a second group practice.

Practise on case studies

Health, social care and education professionals can practise applying the TOM scoring in different ways. One approach that we would suggest is as follows.

An individual presents a case study of a patient/client/student well known to him/her. He/she should outline:

- age

- medical/diagnostic aetiology

- the condition, detailing severity and complicating factors and results of any formal assessments

- what the patient/client/student is able/unable to do for himself/herself and the assistance they require

- the social circumstances, social disadvantage and participation at home, school, work and in recreation. What autonomy or control over their own life do they have?

- their emotional state and general wellbeing

- the emotional status and general wellbeing of their carer if this is relevant

- the priorities for the planned intervention
- agree whether to use the core or an adapted scale.

All other participants may ask questions to the presenter until they feel comfortable to rate the case using the TOM independently. When everyone has completed scoring, they should share the scores with the group. The participants who have attributed scores at variance with the group should explain their reasoning. It is unlikely that all those involved will agree on exactly the same score. The objective of these first attempts is to achieve agreement by 80% of the group within one whole point with subsequent attempts demonstrating increased agreement. This approach to training has been found to improve familiarity and understanding of the scale. It helps participants to identify the behaviours needed to make a decision using the TOM descriptors.

There is evidence that individuals using any rating scale or assessment can 'drift' from the specified approach and thus it is useful to regularly practise rating patients with colleagues. This could be undertaken every 2–3 months at a team meeting.

Please refer to page 17 for information about a website which can be used to share and practise rating (Medshr).

Second training session

The second session, which follows the same format as the first, allows the group to share any difficulties they have experienced in applying the TOM. Team rating of cases can resolve difficulties and facilitate accurate rating between team members. The second session should require individuals to undertake the description and scoring of patient/ client/student within a 10-minute period. A reliability check can be conducted in this session, if required. Aim to be within .5 of each other.

Learning prompt sheet

This section is a summary to support your practice in using TOMs.

Impairment

Each team member should rate the severity of the presentation of the disorder as it affects the person's capacities (*for their age*) in their specific area (e.g., gross motor skills, physical deficit, language, cognitive, psychological disorder).

Very Severe	Severe	Severe/ Moderate	Moderate	Mild	No Impairment
0/0.5	1/1.5	2/2.5	3/3.5	4/4.5	5

Activity

Activity is concerned with what someone can do. It is the ability to execute tasks and/or limitations on actions of an individual indicating the level of dependence and independence. It concerns the degree of abnormality (as compared to someone of the same age, gender and culture) in terms of difference from the norm of what someone undertakes. Consider limitations, the person's capabilities and their performance on an activity. Each team member should rate the degree to which a person can perform a task/function *at an age-appropriate level* (e.g., mobility, dexterity, communication, self-feeding, learning, independence, appropriateness of emotional responses, behaviour).

Unable to perform task/totally dependant on others/no awareness of surroundings	Assists/co-operates but burden of task falls on carers/awareness of surroundings	Can undertake some part of task but needs a high level of support to complete/some interaction with environment	Can undertake task/function/interaction in familiar situation but needs some verbal/physical assistance at other times	Requires some minor assistance occasionally or extra time to complete task	Age-appropriately independent/able to function/perform task/interacts with environment appropriately
0/0.5	1/1.5	2/2.5	3/3.5	4/4.5	5

Participation

The whole team should rate the amount of social functioning of the individual within a social context that is: ability to make choices and have control over their lives/environment; self-awareness and confidence; integration into age-appropriate activities; achievement of potential. This dimension reflects the capabilities of the patient/client as well as the environment and those in the environment.

Isolated, no control over environment, no relationships, unable to exercise choice, 'too protected'/total control in family	Very limited choices, little control over life, some awareness of self within environment, very abnormal role/control	Able to make some choices, able to access nonintegrated facilities, moderately abnormal role in family/environment	Some supported integration, achievement of potential with encouragement, some control over life, some normal control/role	Mostly confident, occasionally some restriction in integration or lack of confidence	Integrated, valued and autonomous in family and society
0/0.5	1/1.5	2/2.5	3/3.5	4/4.5	5

Wellbeing

The team should rate the degree of upset affecting the person/carer (2 scores). See note after the table.

Severe consistent distress, complete detachment – no appropriate emotions	Severe consistent distress frequently experienced; mainly detached	Moderate consistent distress, severe occasional distress, frequent detachment	Moderate distress frequently experienced, often inappropriately detached	Distress occasionally experienced, occasional inappropriate detachment	No inappropriate distress/ detachment
0/0.5	1/1.5	2/2.5	3/3.5	4/4.5	5

*Do not try to attribute distress to any aspect of the person's life or difficulties. Rate this overall even if you think the degree of upset is related to some extraneous issue, e.g., finances/housing, etc.

Case studies/practising

Practising rating individuals with a range of difficulties will assist you to become familiar with the TOM approach and internalize some of the principles. First, you will be able to rate patients more quickly but, more importantly, it will improve your reliability, giving stability to judgements.

We have entered an agreement with MedShr, a fully GMC-, HIPAA- and GDPR-compliant clinical case discussion app and web platform for verified healthcare professionals. MedShr is the easiest and safest way to discuss and share clinical cases and connect with other healthcare professionals and students alike to share knowledge and learn from each other in a private, professional network. There is a 'Therapy Outcome Measure Rehabilitation Discussion Group' on MedShr which you can join by using this link: https://medshr.it/toms

In this group you can identify case studies appropriate for your area of work so that you can practise your rating skills. Furthermore, you can add your own case studies or discuss key topics and issues that are causing you concern with regards to TOM ratings. Creating a case takes just a few minutes. All case studies must be anonymized to ensure they comply with data regulations.

If you have any questions or would like some help getting started, the MedShr team will be pleased to assist you (contact@medshr.net).

3 Data collection

What information should be collected?

A suggested data collection form can be found on page 21. This can be used as a template for adaptation for your own hard copy or electronic form.

Some additional information may be desirable according to the analyses that you wish to undertake. For example, if you wish to examine outcome measures by individual members of staff, it will be necessary to have a space for this information. If you wish to analyze the information on outcomes related to the duration of treatment/ episode of care, you will need to fill in the dates and duration on completion when the final score is detailed.

It is essential that the details of these requirements are agreed between the members of the team as it is important that data are collected consistently by all staff members. To ensure that all those using the system comply consistently over time, it is suggested that local arrangements be written down and included in the induction pack.

ICD codes

Most reports of outcome measures are grouped according to the impairment/disorder, e.g., outcome reports related to people with progressive neurological disease receiving physiotherapy or individuals with dementia receiving occupational therapy. This is one reason for using the ICD 10/11 codes. If you are analyzing data locally, you may wish to amend the aetiologies or impairment codes to suit those already mandated by your computer system. National Health Service systems already integrate ICD 10/11 codes.

The purpose of collecting the diagnosis is to capture the particular disorder that relates to the current period of treatment. That is not to say that there are no other co-existing medical conditions. For example, an individual with Parkinson's disease may suffer a stroke, which results in multifactorial neurological conditions, or an individual with learning difficulties may suffer a head injury. Co-existing conditions should be detailed as such.

In trials, we found that many patients have more than one impairment. These can be coded on the TOM data collection sheet or within your system (if you have specified this requirement) as Code 1 or Code 2. Code 1 should reflect the primary impairment requiring intervention and associated with the referral at this time. If a multidisciplinary team is working on the same impairments (e.g., those associated with rehabilitation after stroke), then it may be appropriate to agree the ratings together. However, where different members of the team are taking particular responsibility for intervention with one aspect so, for example, the speech and language therapist may be focusing on dysphagia, then it would be relevant for her/him to use the dysphagia impairment and activity scales separately to the impairment and activity scales used by other members of the team. Being generic, the participation and wellbeing scales would be the same and determined by the team together.

TOM ratings

The first assessment of the patient/client, or when the therapist has sufficient information to begin active treatment, should be identified with an 'A' beside the first score that you note on a patient/client. The initial assessment of an episode of care may be arrived at after the first appointment or first few appointments which are frequently used to gather case history information, undertake assessments, and agree goals, but it should be entered prior to beginning any active intervention.

An 'I' score denotes an 'Intermediate score' when you are reviewing the patient/client or changing the episode of care. There may be several 'I' scores if the client/patient/student is receiving long-term service involvement.

'F' should identify the 'final' score of an episode of care or at discharge and should be accompanied with the discharge code identifying the reason for discharge (see page 6).

Sometimes clients only need to be seen once, and on such occasions assessment and outcome can be rated within one session. This might be because the client requires advice or the provision of a piece of equipment. In this instance, it may be appropriate to rate the person at the start of the session and then at the end of the session. Record these ratings as 'admission' and 'final' respectively, and use the relevant discharge code.

However, if you are going to follow up such a case with a review appointment or a telephone checkup, record how the client presented at the start as an admission and then at the end of the initial session as an 'intermediate' rating. Then, when you do a follow-up review, the final outcome can be rated according to how the client presents at the review appointment or following the conversation on the telephone.

To comply with the philosophy of this approach, which is to reflect the therapist's clinical judgement, it is allowable to amend this initial assessment score if subsequent information is elicited that would modify the clinical view. For example, if a patient/client reports that they are getting out and about frequently and have kept up with their friends but it turns out later that they do not go out at all and are isolated the therapist may wish to lower the 'A' score for Participation.

Discharge/end of episode codes

Do not forget to add the discharge code, as you may want to analyze data associated with clients who have completed their treatment separately from those who were discharged because of being transferred elsewhere before treatment completion.

If the patient/client, at any stage, has an intervening illness/event and needs a new course of therapy, a discharge code can be used and a new 'A' score should be used to identify this.

Much of this data will already be collected in the computer system used in your department. The essential additional data fields that you need to add to your system are detailed in the table below.

Therapist identity/code :
Patient/client Identity :
(Name or Code Number)
N.B. This information is for local use and will be removed before the Data Sheet leaves the Service

Employing Authority :_____

Locality :_____

Profession :   Speech and Language Therapy, Physiotherapy,Occupational Therapy, Rehabilitation Nursing, Hearing Therapists

Patient/client/Client Details

Age at Entry

Date of Birth : ____/____/_____   **Carer :**_____(person rated)
                 dd   mm   yyyy

Aetiology Code 1 :_____ _____   **Aetiology Code 2 :**_____ _____

Impairment Code 1 :_____ _____   **TOM scale used :**

Impairment Code 2 :_____ _____   **TOM scale used :**

Ratings

Code**	Impairment Code 1 Code 2		Activity	Social Participation	Well-being Patient/client Carer		Date Rated
A-							
I-							

**A = Admission to therapy, First rating : I = Intermediate ratings (when placed at the first entry it denotes previous interventions from therapy) F = Final rating.

Number of Contacts :_____ **Total time :** _____hrs_____mins **Discharge Code** _____

Comments :_____
_____
_____
_____

Please send this form to your key worker for checking and data entry.

Figure 3.1 Example Template Data Collection Form

*aetiology= ICD 10/11 code

It should be noted that some adapted scales do not follow the standard structure. For example, with the AAC adapted scale, there are five sub-domains of 'impairment' and with the Hearing Therapy/Aural Rehabilitation scale, you collect two ratings for the impairment and activity domains (aided and unaided). If using these scales, you will need to adapt your data collection template to enable this information to be recorded. Please refer to the individual adapted scales for details about the information collected.

4 Analyzing the data

Outcomes data become useful when they can be analyzed and used to inform practice. How the data are analyzed will depend on the questions being asked and the audience requiring the information. For example, if you wish to review the information collected about an individual service user for the purposes of informing your clinical decision making and sharing information about their outcomes with them, this will be very different from reviewing the outcomes of all individuals accessing a service in order to inform service design and development. Additionally, you will need different information in reports to commissioners of services. Detailed information about data analysis is available in the third edition of *Therapy Outcome Measures for Rehabilitation Professionals* (Enderby & John, 2015), including using this information for benchmarking (Chapter 2) and examples of how to present TOM data in a way that is accessible to service users (Chapter 5). Here we will focus on how to go about a basic analysis for a group of service users and how to present the information. We will also touch on things to consider if you have the option of setting up a data collection system to enable you to carry out a more detailed analysis of your data.

Analyzing change over time

Once you have been using the TOM for a while with a number of service users, you can begin to analyze the change over time associated with an intervention. In order to do so, you will need to have a sufficient number of individuals with ratings both at the start and end of an episode of care. It is advisable to conduct analysis on no fewer than six service users for any given cohort in order to provide you with a sufficient amount of data from which to begin to evaluate, and to minimize the risks of individuals being identifiable from any reports you produce.

There are different approaches that can be taken to compare scores at the start of an episode of care with the end of an episode of care for a group of service users.

Reporting on the direction of change

You may choose to calculate the proportion of the individuals whose scores have increased, stayed the same, or decreased by 0.5 or more between the start and the end of the intervention for each domain of the TOM. For example:

TOM domain	% of individuals whose scores have increased	% of individuals whose scores have stayed the same	% of individuals whose scores have decreased
Impairment	70	20	10
Activity	80	5	15
Participation	65	15	20
Wellbeing	70	15	15
Carer wellbeing	55	25	20

Reporting on the average amount of change

Another approach is to calculate the average start score, the average final score and the average amount of change for the group of service users. For example:

TOM domain	Average start of episode TOM	Average end of episode TOM	Average change
Impairment	2.6	3.57	0.97
Activity	2.65	3.52	0.87
Participation	2.75	3.09	0.34
Wellbeing	3.16	3.67	0.51
Carer wellbeing	3.03	4.17	1.14

A statistical note

The TOM collects ordinal data: data that have a sense of order but for which we cannot be sure that the distances between the consecutive values are equal. Usually, such data should use nonparametric statistics; however, it is now generally agreed that some ordinal data is less 'qualitative' than other data, and that it is reasonable to treat it as interval data and calculate means and medians, as there is sufficient definition to help people perceive the different points on the scale in the same way.

Presenting the information in a report

There are various issues to consider when presenting information in a report:

Providing a visual representation of the information: In some situations, a table of data will be sufficient, but you may find it useful to present the information in an alternative format, such as a bar chart or a pie chart. This will depend on the purpose of the report you are producing and who you are presenting it to.

Writing an accompanying narrative: It is important to provide context to the data in reports to ensure that the data are informative. For example, if you are working with individuals with progressive conditions, it will be important to explain to your audience that maintaining/sustaining a level of functioning and/or wellbeing is a good outcome for this client group. It may also be appropriate to comment on factors such as the proportion of clients that did not complete the episode of care, or changes to staffing or skill mix that can account for any changes in data trends. Providing a narrative will help to ensure that your data are seen in context and interpreted appropriately.

Avoid jargon: Depending on your audience, it may not be appropriate to use terms such as 'impairment' or 'participation', or you may need to explain what these mean. It may be helpful to annex a short summary of the TOM to any reports generated for audiences that are not familiar with the tool.

Using an electronic system to support a more sophisticated analysis of the data

A simple analysis of your data can be achieved using a spreadsheet but most services are now required to collect data associated with their service on a particular computerized data collection system which can also assist with analysis. Adding the fields to the database would allow you to collect and analyze your TOM data and should not be problematic. But it is important to ensure you are clear about how you wish to use your data and the reports you require before discussing your needs with the IT specialists in your facility. In this chapter we detail a basic analysis of the TOM data but you may wish to develop a reporting system that is a little more sophisticated. For example, you might want to look at the severity of cases entering treatment and whether this varies by age. You could then assess whether you are only being referred cases that have a certain degree of severity and review whether clients with less severe difficulties are not being afforded access to your service. For this you would need to ensure that you can relate your outcome data to the age of your clients. Another area of interest may be associated with determining the number of cases with a particular condition making a change positively, negatively or remaining static in different domains.

Furthermore, you may wish to look at the outcome at the time of discharge from your service and whether the intensity or duration of the intervention is similar to that recommended in efficacy studies, or as compared to other services. In this case you would need to ensure that you collect information on the numbers of times that you see your clients and over what period of time they have received treatment in addition to the TOM scores.

Give some thought to the questions the data will help you answer and ensure that you are collecting all data that would be needed to allow this. The data collection forms that we have used in our studies are detailed on page 21.

5 Frequently asked questions

What happens if I see my patient/client only once?

For an outcome to be measured, you need to be able to make two assessments to assess the change engendered by the intervention. This usually involves more than one appointment to ensure outcomes are reflected. At the first appointment you will often undertake formal or informal assessments, provide advice and may recommend an intervention such as equipment provision or particular exercise. You need to have contact again to determine the impact your input has made. Thus the TOM, like any other outcome measure, needs two ratings. However, if you can make two TOM ratings following one session, then do so. For example, a therapist may assess and advise and/or provide an aid or adaptation that can be classed as an intervention. The intervention can be advising on a strategy, such as modified diet, coordination or sequencing of activities, aids or adaptations. This may result in an immediate change in function or socialization and should be captured in the TOM rating. Some assessment and advisory services undertake an audit of their services by contacting a random sample of clients a few weeks later, by phone or in person, to re-evaluate using the TOM for a second time.

What do I do if I see the patient/client only for assessment?

An outcome measure is used to record the impact of an intervention. The TOM is rated once an intervention is planned and treatment goals are set even if this is the provision of advice. A second rating is made when the episode of intervention is complete. Do not carry out a TOM rating if you are only completing an assessment and do not expect this to lead to anything such as advice or provision of equipment and you do not expect to have further input unless you want descriptive data on all those using your service. Please see response to question above if you are seeing the individual for assessment and advice.

What do I do if I do not see the carer?

The carer wellbeing rating is optional and should reflect the level of concern, anxiety or frustration experienced by the carer at the start and end of intervention. It is usually used if you are providing direct input to the carer or when you expect to have an impact on carer wellbeing. If you are not intervening with the carer then you will not need to rate carer wellbeing.

How do I choose the ICD code for the aetiology or the appropriate TOM scale when a patient/client has more than one?

Using an ICD code will help if you want to compare your data with other services as it will ensure that you are comparing like with like. You should use the ICD code to reflect the medical condition/diagnosis (codes for all aetiologies can be accessed online). The code associated with the reason for referral can be entered as the first code (1) (see page 21 for an example of the data entry form). A co-existing condition (to indicate, for example, if someone with a learning difficulty may have a fracture or someone with Parkinson's disease might have a stroke) is entered by coding the accompanying aetiology as ICD second code (2). If there are multiple aetiologies, use the ICD code to indicate their presence. Individuals with more than one aetiology will often require intervention over a longer duration and possibly more frequently.

What do I do if there is more than one disorder?

You should rate the impairment necessitating the intervention.   However, if there is more than one disorder requiring intervention, rate the primary disorder first under impairment 1, the other under impairment 2.

The aetiology is the underlying medical condition, e.g., stroke or dementia, whereas the impairment reflects the therapy diagnosis, e.g., dysphasia or cognitive disorder. Sometimes, of course, they are the same!

How do I rate activity when there is more than one disorder?

Activity concerns the overall performance/independence of the individual in, for example, communication, walking and activities of daily living. Rate the individual's overall and general performance. Do not rate what the person is *capable* of doing, rate what they *are* doing overall. If it is important for you to record a specific activity, then record it separately, e.g., you may wish to record severity and impact of dysphasia separately from overall stroke. You can record a second disorder code to indicate an accompanying disorder, so you will know there is a co-existing problem that could have influenced the final outcome (e.g., challenging behaviour and dyspraxia).

What do I do if there is no adapted scale for a condition?

You can use the TOM core scale (page 55) to indicate the severity of the impairment, limitation in activity, social participation and level of wellbeing of the individual and their carer when relevant.

What happens if my patient/client has variability in performance?

Patients/clients can vary in their capability to perform a task and their ability to sustain that performance. You need to make a judgement on the level of performance that the individual can achieve and sustain for most of the time. Rate the prevalent performance. For example, if an activity is observed very occasionally or only first thing in the morning, that shows capability, but you need to rate the overall performance. The aim of your therapy may be to increase the prevalence of the behaviour the person is capable of and if this is achieved then the improved consistency of the performance can be reflected at the next review.

What do I do if my patient/client has a deteriorating condition?

The TOM will show the deterioration in the impairment dimension. However, interventions may help the individual to sustain activity and participation for a time. Counselling may help support the individual emotionally and can be reflected in the wellbeing dimension. Rating on the TOM may help you to identify how long an individual can sustain his/her activity and quality of life while the disease progresses. A palliative care scale is now available as one of the adapted scales.

How do I rate patients/clients who use environmental aids or augmentative communication?

Please find an adaptation of the TOM specifically for this purpose. You need to make a rating about how the person is managing when referred and subsequently to reflect the difference in ability when their aid/equipment is being used. It is desirable to re-rate when the aid/equipment has been in use for some time to reflect whether it has made a difference to the client's independence and wellbeing.

What do I do if I transfer the patient/client to another clinician?

If transferring within your service, you should provide an intermediate rating 'I' reflecting the situation before you hand over to the other clinician. However, if the client is being transferred to another service you will need to do a final rating 'F' and choose the discharge code of 'transferred' which indicates that the therapy was not complete. Suggested discharge codes are detailed on page 6.

Do I rate depression under 'impairment' or 'wellbeing'?

You need to decide why you are seeing the individual. If the individual is clinically depressed, then you would record that under aetiology, and then rate the impairment that corresponds to their condition, for example, anxiety. If the individual is low in spirit because his/her mood is affected by another condition, then rate the degree of emotional disturbance in the wellbeing dimension.

Should the carer wellbeing be completed by the carers themselves?

TOMs is a clinician-reported outcome measure, meaning that the rating made for each of the domains – including carer wellbeing – reflects the clinician's professional judgement. Nevertheless, it is best practice to gather information from assessments, referral information, observation and other reports as well as determining the service users' and their carers' views on levels of impairment, activity, participation and wellbeing, and to use this information to inform the TOM.

When you are rating participation and wellbeing, is this specific to a specific condition?

No, it has been found to be difficult to attribute a particular level of participation or wellbeing to a specific condition – so these levels reflect the individual's overall participation and wellbeing.

Is it valid for different therapists to rate a patient during an episode of care?

Yes, if they know how to do TOMs and have checked their reliability.

How do I score wellbeing when the patient is unconscious/semi-conscious?

It would not be appropriate to score wellbeing in this situation. Record this as not assessed N/A.

When should I rate a young child?

"When using TOMs with young children with Down Syndrome, I am unsure when to do the first rating. I typically meet the family when the child is 6 months old for an initial assessment. At this point, the child tends to be developing in line with their peers. Delays in expressive language and speech may become apparent between 12 and 18 months of age. Should we be capturing where they are at 6 months old or where they are when they began to show an impairment?"

The TOM approach requires you to rate the person (child) compared to another without the condition but of the same age, gender and culture. Most infants rate quite high initially as, of course, they are being compared with infants who are totally dependent and their difficulty is not exposed till later in their development. This can give the appearance that the child is getting worse over time, but this trajectory will be the same as other children with the same condition. That is why it is useful to collect data identifying the underlying condition, in this case, Down Syndrome.

What should I do if someone leaves half way through treatment?

If the individual does not complete their therapy, you should complete the final rating reflecting how they presented the last time that you worked with them and use the appropriate discharge code (see page 6).

When we start to use the TOM, should we retrospectively rate all of the individuals on our caseload?

If your notes are sufficiently detailed for you to retrospectively record the TOM rating at the beginning of treatment then you can do this. The alternative is to only start using the TOM with new referrals.

Please advise what to do if/when a patient dies in terms of scoring.

If the person dies during an active episode of care and if the therapist feels they know the patient sufficiently well to rate the person based on the last interaction then rate reflecting that situation. However, if not then leave as NA – Not assessed. Do not forget to note the reason for discharge was death. You can use reasons for discharge as a filter when doing your data analysis.

Can our therapy assistants/technical instructors use the TOMs independently?

Therapy assistants/technical instructors who have received TOMs training and are familiar with the principles and scales of the TOMs, having scored up patients/clients regularly and established good agreement/reliability may use the TOMs independently. It is advised that reliability checks are undertaken regularly (approximately once per month) and that colleagues are aware of who within the service to approach with any queries or concerns when using TOMs. Studies have shown that some therapy assistants/ technical instructors can experience particular difficulty differentiating between the domains of 'impairment' and 'activity', and it is therefore suggested that it is helpful to focus on this during local training sessions and ongoing inter-rater reliability checks.

How can we get permission to upload the TOMS forms we use for each individual for their electronic clinical notes?

Permission is granted on page 215 of the 2015 edition: *'It is important to acknowledge the authors and the full publication reference to comply with copyright'*

Can I start using TOMs with patients halfway through their treatment?

Yes, but to help your analysis it is probably best to indicate a new episode of care or intermediate score to indicate that this was not the beginning of treatment.

What should I do if a patient receives a new formal diagnosis (e.g., Aspergers Spectrum Disorder) versus onset of a new condition?

If you need to change the focus of your intervention because of this new information then you will need to open a new episode of care using the adapted scale that is most appropriate. You will need to change the medical diagnostic coding on your data collection form.

What should I do if I do not know how the patient is participating or their state of wellbeing because they are an infant, too ill or unconscious?

If you do not have sufficient information or it would be inappropriate to reflect participation or well-being due to particular circumstances then do not guess! Complete data collection by using NA – not assessed.

6 Do you want to develop or adapt a TOM scale?

You may wish to develop or to adapt a TOM scale for a particular service or specific client group. If you do please read on.

Before you start: Make sure that you have understood the principles of the domains as specified in Enderby and John (2015). Review the 68 adapted scales contained in this book. Is there one that can be modified slightly?

Is there a real need for an adapted scale? Don't forget that for clients with conditions of very low incidence or prevalence and for whom there is no appropriate adapted scale you can use the core scale.

Adapting a scale: You may feel that adapting some of the terminology in the scale to fit with the language you use in your service would help with the understanding and agreement amongst your therapists. Before you do this you should:

- discuss possible changes with your colleagues
- send a copy of your amendments to Pam Enderby (PE) or Alex John (AJ) (contact details: see page viii) for them to check that they are in line with the principles of TOMs
- if the amendments are minor they may be authorized for use straight away
- if the amendments are more major, please read on.

Developing a new scale

Make sure you understand the principles of the TOMs and what is included in each of the domains.

Remember that the aim of the adapted scale is to assist you and colleagues working with the same client group to come to the same decision with regard to abilities and difficulties of the individual.

Inspect some of the adapted scales similar to the client group you are considering.

Discuss with other professionals working with the client group that you are considering how you can develop the descriptors. Sometimes it is helpful to do this together. It is usually easier to describe the descriptors for scale points 0, 1, 4 and 5 before attempting descriptors 2 and 3. Describing what we call 'moderate' is always difficult!

You and your colleagues should try to use this early draft of the scale to rate those clients from the particular client group. Identify any lack of clarity and discuss whether further descriptions would help. Remember that the descriptors are 'best fit' – thus the client may not have all of the behaviours or challenges outlined in the description but this description describes them better than another. It is useful to pilot the use of this with clients known to have behaviours across a range of the scale.

Following a trial of the modified description you should send it to PE or AJ (authors) for them to check that the scale is in line with the principles of the TOMs.

If all is well, then we suggest that you practise using this adapted scale by rating a number of clients, both individually and with your colleagues, to see whether any further minor amendments need to be made. Repeat the process. This iterative approach will help you become familiar with the descriptions and their 'best fit' for the clients in that group.

Once you are satisfied with the wording (validity) of the wording of the adapted scale you should go forward with a reliability trial.

Checking reliability

Checking reliability is important as it represents the extent to which the adapted scale is understood consistently and that the data you collect are a correct representation. Just a reminder: **intra-rater** reliability is the degree of agreement among repeated administrations of a diagnostic test performed by the same rater. To do this you will need to prepare some case histories with sufficient information for the TOM to be carried out by a number of therapists, e.g., six. Ask them to rate these cases and ask them to rate them again a couple of weeks later. Obviously, they should not keep a copy of their first scores! You are trying to find out whether your adapted scale helps them to be consistent over time.

Another reminder: **inter-rater reliability** examines the extent to which those who use the scale assign the same or very close scores to the same variable. We would suggest that you get a group of therapists, preferably a minimum of six, with experience with the relevant client group and who are familiar with the TOMs, to meet together. Each one should describe a case, stating the behaviours using each of the dimensions (impairment, activity, participation and wellbeing). Ask the group to rate the case using the new adapted scale, without collusion. Check agreement of rating on 10 cases. At first, you would expect each therapist to be within one point of each other. After practice they should be getting within .5 of each other.

If you are unable to get a group of therapists together you may want to share an anonymized case history with each therapist by email which they can rate. The lead therapist should check agreement.

1. Count the number of ratings in agreement within .5 of each other.
2. Count the total number of ratings.
3. Divide the total by the number in agreement to get a fraction.
4. Convert to a percentage to represent the percentage of agreement.

You could undertake a Cohen's kappa coefficient (κ) which is a statistic which measures inter-rater agreement for qualitative (categorical) items. It has been developed to take account of the possibility that, due to their uncertainty, raters are likely to guess on at least some variables. Because of this it is thought to be a more robust measure than simple percent agreement calculation.

It is possible that you will find that you will need to add or subtract some phrases from your adapted scale as they are being interpreted differently by different raters.

Keep in touch with PE and AJ who can provide further advice if required. You may be asked whether you would agree to the scale that you have developed being included in the next edition of the book. Your leadership on this piece of work would be acknowledged.

Note. It is advisable to have the following header on your adapted scale:

Therapy Outcome Measure Adapted Scale (*add client group*) – in development

The individual does not have to have each feature mentioned in the descriptor. It is a best fit description, i.e., does this description fit the individual better than the other one. Use 0.5 to indicate if the individual is slightly better or worse than the descriptor. Consider as appropriate for age, gender and culture.

To comply with copyright please add the following footer:

Therapy Outcome Measure Adapted Scale for [...] in development in line with principles detailed in: Enderby P. & John A. (2015). *Therapy Outcome Measures for Rehabilitation Professionals*, 3rd edition. Guildford: J&R Press.

7 Use of the TOM by the Royal College of Speech and Language Therapists

Case study: The RCSLT Online Outcome Tool

Background

In the UK, The Royal College of Speech and Language Therapists (RCSLT) has established a programme of work on outcome measurement to support its members with improving the collection of data to reflect the impact of speech and language therapy for individuals with speech, language, communication and swallowing needs. Following the introduction of outcomes-based commissioning in some parts of the UK, it was recognized that the speech and language therapy (SLT) profession needed to have more objective evidence of the impact of SLT services.

On recognizing that the development of an outcome tool would take a significant number of years, the RCSLT set about identifying an existing outcome measure that could be used by the SLT profession to gather consistent data. Following an appraisal of available outcome measurement tools against a set of criteria agreed by members, the TOM was identified as the best fit for purpose at this time, acknowledging that the adoption of the TOM was a starting point for the profession's journey on outcome measurement.

One of the barriers to using outcome measurement tools as reported by members of the SLT profession was the limited availability of digital systems to record and analyze the data. The RCSLT commissioned Different Class Solutions Ltd to develop an online data collection tool to support with collecting, collating and reporting on the TOM data. The development of the RCSLT Online Outcome Tool (ROOT) has been undertaken in collaboration with RCSLT officers, Pam Enderby and speech and language therapists involved in a pilot.

How does the ROOT support collecting and analyzing TOM data?

SLT services that do not have local electronic systems to support collection of their TOM data can input data directly into the ROOT for each individual they are working with. This enables them to record the information in a systematic way at various points in the individual's care. Figure 7.1 shows a screenshot of the ROOT.

Services that can digitally record their TOM data in a local system/database can also share their data with the ROOT by extracting it from their local system and transferring it in bulk. To facilitate this, Different Class Solutions developed a bespoke solution.

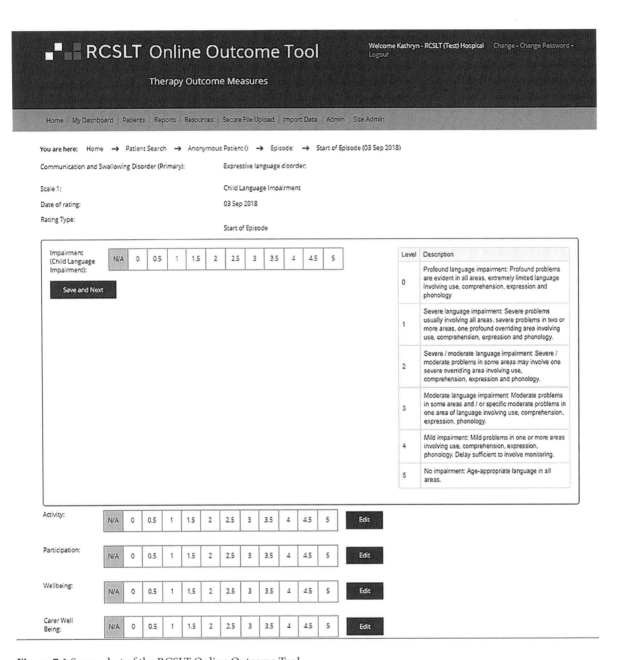

Figure 7.1 Screenshot of the RCSLT Online Outcome Tool.

Both methods of data collection enable SLTs to access reports on their TOM data. This includes reports showing change over time in association with SLT interventions for individual service users (Figures 7.2 and 7.3) for the domains of impairment, activity, participation and wellbeing and, where appropriate, carer wellbeing.

The ROOT also generates reports for groups of service users. It is possible to

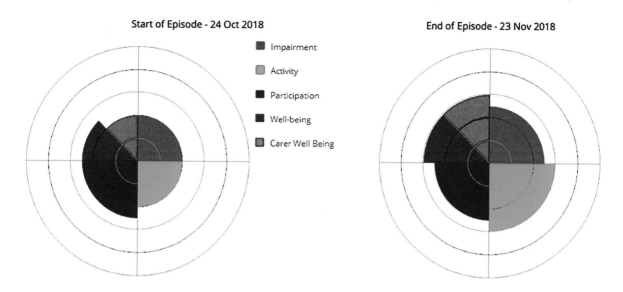

Figure 7.2 A report for an individual service user showing the TOM scores for the domains of impairment, activity, participation, wellbeing and carer wellbeing at the start and end of an episode of care.

apply a number of parameters to the reports to enable the data to be interrogated at the appropriate level for various purposes. For example, if a service was interested in the difference between dysphagia outcomes for individuals with different underlying conditions, it is possible to drill down to look at this; Figure 7.4 shows a report for 322

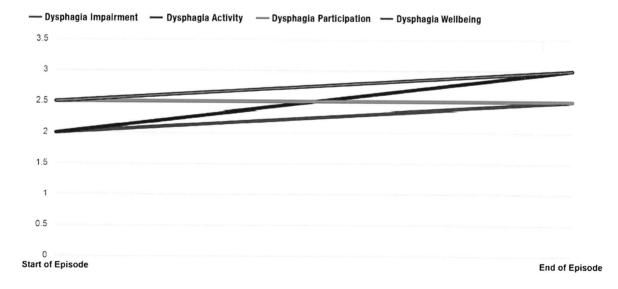

Figure 7.3 A report for an individual service user showing the changes in TOM scores over the course of an episode of care for the domains of impairment, activity, participation and wellbeing.

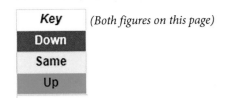

Key
Down
Same
Up

(Both figures on this page)

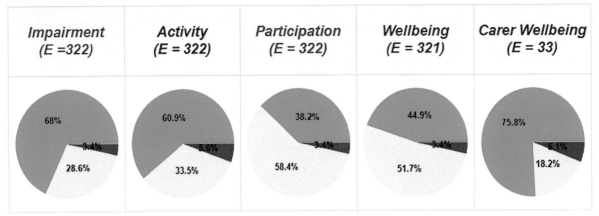

Impairment (E =322)	Activity (E = 322)	Participation (E = 322)	Wellbeing (E = 321)	Carer Wellbeing (E = 33)
68% / 3.4% / 28.6%	60.9% / 5.6% / 33.5%	38.2% / 3.4% / 58.4%	44.9% / 3.4% / 51.7%	75.8% / 6.1% / 18.2%

Figure 7.4 A report generated by the ROOT showing the percentage of individuals with dysphagia in association with stroke whose TOM scores have increased (green), stayed the same (yellow) and decreased (red) over the course of an episode of care for the domains of impairment, activity, participation and wellbeing.

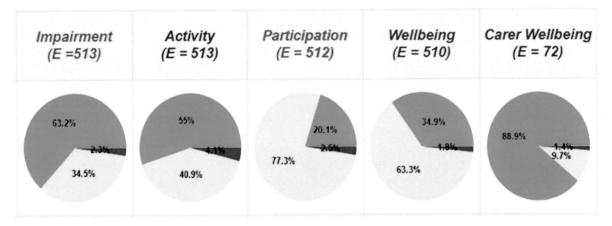

Impairment (E =513)	Activity (E = 513)	Participation (E = 512)	Wellbeing (E = 510)	Carer Wellbeing (E = 72)
63.2% / 2.3% / 34.5%	55% / 4.1% / 40.9%	20.1% / 2.6% / 77.3%	34.9% / 1.8% / 63.3%	88.9% / 1.4% / 9.7%

Figure 7.5 A report generated by the ROOT showing the percentage of individuals dysphagia in association with dementia whose TOM scores have increased (green), stayed the same (yellow) and decreased (red) over the course of an episode of care for the domains of impairment, activity, participation and well-being.

service users with dysphagia in association with stroke and Figure 7.5 shows a report for 513 services uses with dysphagia in association with dementia.

Other parameters that can be applied to the ROOT include age and gender. It is also possible to filter the data by the severity of the primary impairment, to differentiate between individuals with progressive and nonprogressive conditions, and to look specifically at groups of service users that have co-occurring conditions.

The reports available on the ROOT present the information in a variety of ways, to accommodate the various audiences; some provide a high level analysis of the trends in the data (e.g., Figures 7.4 and 7.5) while others provide a detailed breakdown of the average amount of change (Figure 7.6).

Service A	Average Type	Impairment			Activity			Participation			Wellbeing			Carer Wellbeing		
		Start	End	Change	Start	End	Change	Start	End	Change	Start	End	Change	Start	End	Change
All Toms Scales Episodes: (2551) Patients: (2551)	Mean	2.66	3.58	0.92	2.72	3.57	0.85	2.87	3.27	0.4	3.18	3.74	0.55	2.99	4.13	1.15
	Median	2.5	2.5	1	2.5	2.5	1	2.5	3	1	2.5	3	1	2.5	3	1
Aphasia/Dysphasia Episodes: (221) Patients: (221)	Mean	2.22	2.98	0.75	2.39	3.16	0.77	2.32	3.07	0.76	2.76	3.49	0.73	2.43	3.35	1
	Median	2.5	2.5	1.5	2.5	2.5	1.5	2.5	2.5	1.5	2.5	2.5	0.75	2.5	2.5	0.75
Cognition Episodes: (7) Patients: (7)	Mean	2.64	2.57	-0.07	2.43	2.21	-0.21	2	1.79	-0.21	3	3	0	3.5	4	0.5
	Median	2.5	2.5	0.25	2	2.25	0	2	2	0	2	2	0	2	2	0
Core Scale Episodes: (31) Patients: (31)	Mean	2.52	3	0.48	2.81	3.19	0.39	3.06	3.31	0.24	2.84	3.37	0.53	3.11	3.33	0.17
	Median	2.5	2.5	1	2.25	3	0.75	2.5	3	0.75	2.75	2.75	1	2.75	2.75	1
Dysarthria Episodes: (190) Patients: (190)	Mean	3.45	3.81	0.36	3.77	4.12	0.35	3.59	4.03	0.43	3.59	4.08	0.49	3.16	3.78	0.5
	Median	2.5	2.5	0.5	2.75	3	0.5	2.5	3	1.25	2.75	2.75	1.25	2.75	2.75	1.25
Dysfluency Episodes: (15) Patients: (15)	Mean	2.73	3.2	0.47	2.4	3.13	0.73	3.13	3.73	0.6	2.67	3.47	0.8			
	Median	2.5	3	1	2.25	3.25	1.25	2.5	3.5	1	2.5	4	1.25	2.5	4	1.25
Dysphagia Episodes: (1804) Patients: (1804)	Mean	2.64	3.68	1.04	2.65	3.58	0.93	2.69	3.05	0.36	3.14	3.66	0.52	2.99	4.21	1.25
	Median	2.5	2.5	0.75	2.75	2.5	0.5	2.5	2.5	0.5	2.25	2.25	0.25	2.25	2.25	0.25
Dysphonia Episodes: (283) Patients: (283)	Mean	2.64	3.41	0.78	2.73	3.54	0.81	3.95	4.37	0.42	3.59	4.27	0.68	3.87	4.22	0.11
	Median	2.5	2.75	1.25	2.5	2.5	2	3.25	3.25	1	2.75	3.25	0.75	2.75	3.25	0.75

Figure 7.6 A report generated by the ROOT showing the average TOM scores at the start and end of the episode of care and the average amount of change for the domains of impairment, activity, participation, wellbeing and carer wellbeing for a particular service.

The value of outcome measurement in speech and language therapy

Speech and language therapists involved in the ROOT pilot highlighted the value of being able to report on the data they have collected, both in their everyday working and for the benefit of the service. For SLTs using the TOM in clinical practice, the ROOT reports have enabled them to see, at a glance, the impact of their interventions. For clinical leads and service managers, aggregated reports have been reported as useful in the context of service planning and providing intelligence to key stakeholders, including budget holders and commissioners. Members have also indicated the potential of using the reports to support service improvement and for influencing purposes.

Through using the ROOT, the SLT profession has a growing database of information about the impact of interventions for individuals with speech, language, communication and swallowing difficulties (Enderby & Moyse, 2018). There is the potential for the SLT profession to use this information to drive quality improvement by learning from areas of best practice. Collecting outcome data using a consistent approach across the SLT profession also provides an opportunity to use data to assist with improving public awareness, influencing politicians and campaigning for investment in services.

Reference

Enderby, P. & Moyse, K. (2018). International Classification of Functioning – An approach to outcome measurement. Perspectives of the ASHA Special Interest Groups SIG, 17, Vol. 3(Part 2). American Speech-Language-Hearing Association.

References/Bibliography

TOMs used in research

Ali, K., Gammidge, T., & Waller, D. (2014). Fight like a ferret: A novel approach of using art therapy to reduce anxiety in stroke patients undergoing hospital rehabilitation. *Medical Humanities, 4*(1), 56, LP-60. DOI: 10.1136/medhum-2013-010448

Caldwell, C., Twelvetree, T., & Cox, D. (2015). An evaluation of Therapy Outcome Measures (TOMs) in community rehabilitation. *International Journal of Therapy and Rehabilitation, 22*(7), 310–319.

Dixon, S., Nancarrow, S.A., Enderby, P.M., Moran, A.M., & Parker, S.G. (2015). Assessing patient preferences for the delivery of different community-based models of care using a discrete choice experiment. *Health Expectations, 18*(5), 1204–1214.

Enderby, P. & Moyse, K. (2018). International Classification of Functioning - An Approach to Outcome Measurement. *Perspectives of the ASHA Special Interest Groups, 3*(17), 99–108.

Horton, S., Clark, A., Barton, G., Lane, K., & Pomeroy, V.M. (2016). Methodological issues in the design and evaluation of supported communication for aphasia training: A cluster-controlled feasibility study. *BMJ Open, 6*(4), e011207.

Mitchell, C., Bowen, A., Tyson, S., & Conroy, P. (2017). ReaDySpeech for people with dysarthria after stroke: Protocol for a feasibility randomised controlled trial. *Pilot and Feasibility Studies, 4*(1), 25.

Palmer, R., Cooper, C., Enderby, P., Brady, M., Julious, S., Bowen, A., & Latimer, N. (2015). Clinical and cost effectiveness of computer treatment for aphasia post stroke (Big CACTUS): Study protocol for a randomised controlled trial. *Trials, 16*(1), 18. https://doi.org/10.1186/s13063-014-0527-7

Radford, K., Woods, H., Lowe, D., & Rogers, S.N. (2004). A UK multi-centre pilot study of speech and swallowing outcomes following head and neck cancer. *Clinical Otolaryngology & Allied Sciences, 29*(4), 376–381.

Ward, E.C., Bishop, B., Frisby, J., & Stevens, M. (2002) Swallowing outcomes following laryngectomy and pharyngolaryngectomy. *Archives of Otolaryngology Head Neck Surgery, 128*(2), 181–186.

TOMs referenced in articles on outcome measures

Beresford, B.A., Clarke, S., & Maddison, J.R. (2018). Therapy interventions for children with neurodisabilities: A qualitative scoping study of current practice and perceived research needs. *Health Technology Assessment*. DOI: 10.3310/hta22030

Dodd, B. (2005). *Differential Diagnosis and Treatment of Children with Speech Disorder*. John Wiley & Sons.

Enderby, P. (2014). Introducing the therapy outcome measure for AAC services in the context of a review of other measures. *Disability and Rehabilitation: Assistive Technology, 9*(1), 33–40.

Enderby, P. (2014). Use of the extended therapy outcome measure for children with dysarthria. *International Journal of Speech-Language Pathology, 16*(4), 436–444. DOI: 10.3109/17549507.2014.902994

Enderby, P. (2017). Speech pathology as the MasterChef: Getting the right ingredients and stirring the pot. *International Journal of Speech-Language Pathology*, *19*(3), 232–236.

Enderby, P., Ariss, S., Bradburn, M., Ryan, T., & Cambell, M. (2014). Enhancing the efficiency and effectiveness of community-based services for older people: A secondary analysis to inform service delivery. *Clinical Rehabilitation*, *28*(11), 1154.

Gomersall, T., Spencer, S., Basarir, H., Tsuchiya, A., Clegg, J., Sutton, A., & Dickinson, K. (2015). Measuring quality of life in children with speech and language difficulties: A systematic review of existing approaches. *International Journal of Language & Communication Disorders*, *50*(4), 416–435.

Harron, A. & Titterington, J. (2016). Use of outcome measurement by paediatric AHPs in Northern Ireland. *International Journal of Language & Communication Disorders*, *51*(4), 487–492.

Hilari, K., Klippi, A., Constantinidou, F., Horton, S., Penn, C., Raymer, A., & Worrall, L. (2015). An international perspective on quality of life in aphasia: A survey of clinician views and practices from sixteen countries. *Folia Phoniatrica et Logopaedica*, *67*(3), 119–130. DOI: 10.1159/000434748

Hoskin, J. & Garwood, G. (2018). *Discovering Who I am: A Group Resource for Children and Young People Working on Social and Emotional Wellbeing and Identity*. (Chapter 3, Facilitating groups from preparation to evaluation). London: Routledge.

Isaksen, J.K. (2014). 'It really makes good sense': The role of outcome evaluation in aphasia therapy in Denmark. *International Journal of Language & Communication Disorders*, *49*(1), 90–99.

John, A. (2011). Therapy outcome measures: Where are we now? *International Journal of Speech-Language Pathology*, *13*(1), 36–42.

Karlsson, P., Allsop, A., Dee-Price, B.-J., & Wallen, M. (2018). Eye-gaze control technology for children, adolescents and adults with cerebral palsy with significant physical disability: Findings from a systematic review. *Developmental Neurorehabilitation*, *21*(8), 497–505.

Long, A.F., Hesketh, A., Paszek, G., Booth, M., & Bowen, A. (2008). Development of a reliable self-report outcome measure for pragmatic trials of communication therapy following stroke: The Communication Outcome after Stroke (COAST) scale. *Clinical Rehabilitation*, *22*(12), 1083–1094. DOI: 10.1177/0269215508090091

Mackenzie, C., Paton, G., Kelly, S., Brady, M., & Muir, M. (2012). The Living With Dysarthria Group: Implementation and feasibility of a group intervention for people with dysarthria following stroke and family members. *International Journal of Language & Communication Disorders*, *47*(6), 709–724.

McCartney, E. (2017). Measuring communication and participation in children with speech and language disorders. *Developmental Medicine & Child Neurology*, *59*(5), 459–460.

McLeod, S., McCartney, E., & McCormack, J. (2012). What is the construct? https://pureportal.strath.ac.uk/files-asset/14120946/Chapter_22_2_.pdf

Moran, A., Nancarrow, S., Enderby, P., & Bradburn, M. (2012). Are we using support workers effectively? The relationship between patient and team characteristics and support worker utilisation in older people's community-based rehabilitation services in England. *Health & Social Care in the Community*, *20*(5), 537–549.

Rees, J., Muskett, T., Enderby, P., & Stackhouse, J. (2016). Implications of untreated cleft palate in the developing world: Adaptation of an outcome measure. *Folia Phoniatrica et Logopaedica*, *68*(1), 1–9.

Roteno, T. & Ariss, S. (2014) Multidisciplinary team effectiveness in the community-based stroke care services in the UK. *Indonesian Journal of Physical Medicine, 3*, 59-72.

Roulstone, S., John, A., Hughes, A., & Enderby, P. (2004). Assessing the construct validity of the Therapy Outcome Measure for pre-school children with delayed speech and language. *Advances in Speech Language Pathology*, *6*(4), 230–236. DOI: 10.1080/14417040400010181

Saville, R. (2018). Applying the 'East Kent Outcomes System'(EKOS) in music therapy. *APPROACHES: An Interdisciplinary Journal for Music Therapy*, *10*(1).

References related to the development of TOM

Enderby, P. (1992). Outcome measures in speech therapy: Impairment, disability, handicap, and distress. *Health Trends, 24*, 61-64.

Enderby, P. & John, A. (1997). *Therapy Outcome Measures: Speech-Language Pathology*. San Diego/London: Singular.

Enderby, P. & John, A. (1999). Therapy outcome measures in speech and language therapy: Comparing performance between different providers. *International Journal of Language and Communication Disorders*, 34, 417-429.

Enderby, P., John, A., & Petheram B. (1998). *Therapy Outcome Measures: Physiotherapy, Occupational Therapy, Rehabilitation Nursing*. San Diego/London: Singular.

Enderby, P., John, A., Sloan, M., & Petheram, B. (1995). *Outcome Measures in Speech and Language Therapy*. Bristol: Speech and Language Therapy Research Unit.

Enderby, P., John, A., Hughes, A., & Petheram, B. (2000). Benchmarking in rehabilitation: Comparing physiotherapy services. *British Journal of Clinical Governance*, 5(2), 86-92.

Enderby, P., Hughes, A., John, A., & Petheram, B. (2003). Using benchmark data for assessing performance in occupational therapy. *Clinical Governance*, 8(4), 290-295.

Hammerton, J. (2004). An investigation into the influence of age on recovery from stroke with community rehabilitation. PhD Thesis (unpublished), Sheffield University.

John, A. (2005). Comparing outcomes of voice therapy: A benchmarking study using the therapy outcome measure. *Journal of Voice, 19*(1), 114-23.

Marshall, M. (2004). A study to elicit the core components of stroke rehabilitation and the subsequent development of a taxonomy of the therapy process. PhD Thesis, Sheffield University.

World Health Organization (2001). *International Classification of Functioning, Disability and Health (ICF)*. Geneva: WHO.

TOM Scales

Acknowledgements

Developed scales

We would like to acknowledge the assistance of literally hundreds of health, social care and education professionals who have contributed to the development, amendments and adaptations of the Therapy Outcome Measure adapted scales for particular client groups. We sincerely appreciate their contribution. Whilst it is invidious to name a few, there are some who have had substantial influence on the new scales included in this edition.

These include: Joan Murphy and Sally Boa (AAC), Graeme Marsh (Equipment Services), Lyndsay-Jayne Charles (Learning Disability), Julia Johnston (Palliative Care), Sally-Anne Search, Carol Weir, Katie Johnson, Susan Warren, Tracy Parkinton, Hannah Yates and Bernadette Maclagan, Elinor Campbell, Edward Nottingham (Eating Disorders), Heather Hill (Paediatric Dietetics), Emma Hutton (Dementia), Alison Martin (Special Schools), Hilary Lewis (Postnatal Depression, Chronic Pain), Victoria Sleight (Challenging Behaviour and Forensic), Jennifer Reid (Speech and Language Therapy Services), Victoria Bulbeck (Pulmonary Conditions), Gillian Osborne, Lesley Spencer (Podiatry), Lisa Maendl (Head Injury), Jo Rees (Cleft Palate), Sarah Haynes (Tracheostomy). And many, many, more! Sincere apologies if we have left someone out!

Scales in development

Further adapted scales have been developed by specialists in specific topics, used in clinical settings and found to be useful and acceptable but have not as yet been tested rigorously for their inter-rater reliability. These are clearly marked 'scale under development'. Clinicians initiating the development are acknowledged at the end of each as appropriate.

List of Scales

*Reliability is requiring further testing.

New Adapted Scales Fully Tested   193

Scales in Development

TOM Core Scale

Identify descriptor that is 'best fit'. The patient/client does not have to have each feature mentioned. Use 0.5 to indicate if the patient/client is slightly better or worse than a descriptor and as appropriate to age.

Impairment

0 The most severe presentation of this impairment.

1 Severe presentation of this impairment.

2 Severe/moderate presentation.

3 Moderate presentation.

4 Just below normal/mild impairment.

5 No impairment.

Activity

0 Totally dependent/unable to function.

1 Assists/cooperates but burden of task/achievement falls on professional or caregiver.

2 Can undertake some part of task but needs a high level of support to complete.

3 Can undertake task/function in familiar situation but requires some verbal/physical assistance.

4 Requires some minor assistance occasionally or extra time to complete task.

5 Independent/able to function.

Participation

0 **No autonomy, isolated, no social/family life.**

1 **Very limited choices, contact mainly with professionals, no social or family role, little control over life.**

2 **Some integration, value and autonomy in one setting.**

3 **Integrated, valued and autonomous in limited number of settings.**

4 **Occasionally some restriction in autonomy, integration or role.**

5 **Integrated, valued, occupies appropriate role.**

Wellbeing/Distress

0 Severe constant: High and constant levels of distress/upset/concern/frustration/anger/embarrassment/withdrawal/severe depression/or apathy, unable to express or control emotions appropriately.

1 Frequently severe: Moderate distress/upset/concern/frustration/anger/embarrassment/withdrawal/severe depression/or apathy. Becomes concerned easily, requires constant reassurance/support, needs clear/tight limits and structure, loses emotional control easily.

2 Moderate consistent: Distress/upset/concern/frustration/anger/embarrassment/withdrawal/severe depression/or apathy in unfamiliar situations, frequent emotional encouragement and support required.

3 Moderate frequent: Distress/upset/concern/frustration/anger/embarrassment/withdrawal/severe depression/or apathy. Controls emotions with assistance, emotionally dependent on some occasions, vulnerable to change in routine, etc., spontaneously uses methods to assist emotional control.

4 Mild occasional: Distress/upset/concern/frustration/anger/embarrassment/withdrawal/severe depression/or apathy. Able to control feelings in most situations, generally well adjusted/stable (most of the time/most situations), occasional emotional support/encouragement needed.

5 Not inappropriate: Distress/upset/concern/frustration/anger/embarrassment/withdrawal/severe depression/or apathy. Well adjusted, stable and able to cope emotionally with most situations, good insight, accepts and understands own limitations.

Developed Scales

1 Anorexia Nervosa and Bulimia

Identify descriptor that is 'best fit'. The patient/client/student does not have to have each feature mentioned. Use 0.5 to indicate if patient/client/student is slightly better or worse than a descriptor and as appropriate to age.

Impairment

0 On complete bed rest and requiring daily monitoring of all physical observations due to extremely low body weight that presents risk of serious health problems and/or death, refusing all nutrition, persistently attempting to engage in compensatory behaviours* with the aim to induce further weight loss.

1 Severe presentation of Anorexia Nervosa or Bulimia Nervosa. Takes in a minimal amount of nutrition/or expels most nutrition, requires high level of support to engage in eating, and/or regularly engages in a range of compensatory behaviours* with the aim to induce further weight loss.

2 Severe/moderate presentation of Anorexia Nervosa or Bulimia Nervosa. Takes in minimal/moderate amount of nutrition or attempts to expel substantial amount of nutrition, requires moderate level of support to engage in eating, and/or severe/moderate engagement in a range of compensatory behaviours* with the aim to induce further weight loss.

3 Moderate presentation of Anorexia Nervosa or Bulimia Nervosa. Takes in moderate amount of nutrition and makes regular attempts to expel nutrition, requires some regular support to engage in eating, and/or infrequent engagement in a range of compensatory behaviours* with the aim to induce further weight loss.

4 Mild presentation of Anorexia Nervosa or Bulimia Nervosa. Increased awareness of nutritional intake relating to weight control occasional attempt to expel nutrition and/or occasional use of compensatory behaviours*.

5 No evidence of presentation of Anorexia Nervosa or Bulimia Nervosa.

*NB compensatory behaviours include fasting, purging, excessive exercise, laxative abuse, etc.

Activity

0 Supervised nasogastric tube feeding.

1 Supervised use of nutritional supplements and/or artificial nutrition in conjunction with a small amount of oral diet.

2 High level of supervision and support required for many activities, especially those related to eating in order to maintain small oral intake. Strong reliance on professional or caregiver for the preparation of diet and other activities.

3 Some supervision required for many activities, especially those related to eating and for maintenance of oral diet at full portion size. Frequent reliance on professional or caregiver for the preparation of diet.

4 Takes overall responsibility for most activities of daily living, including those related to eating, shopping, preparing, cooking, portioning and eating of an appropriately nutritionally balanced diet. Still requires occasional support, encouragement and direction in these areas of activity.

5 Complete independence in all activities of daily living including shopping, preparing, cooking, portioning and eating of an appropriately nutritionally balanced diet.

Participation

0 Profound difficulty in participating. Complete bed rest, may require frequent restraint. Unable to participate in any social/educational/family role. No social integration.

1 Very limited choices, contact mainly with professionals, no social or family role, little control over life or participation in an inappropriately wide range of settings/activities as a means of compensating for nutritional intake or avoiding stressors. Avoids all social activities involving food and/or drink.

2 Some integration, value in one setting or a very high level of involvement in a broad spectrum of settings/activities as a means of compensating for nutritional intake or avoiding stressors. Avoids most social activities involving food and/or drink.

3 Integrated, valued and autonomous in limited number of settings or a significant level of involvement in multiple settings/activities as a means of compensating for nutritional intake or avoiding stressors. Can tolerate some social activities involving food and drink with some support.

4 Occasionally some restriction in autonomy, integration or role, is able to cope with most social activities involving food and/or drink independently but requires support on some occasions.

5 Integrated in a number of valued appropriate roles. No difficulty in participating. Fully confident and participates in normal activities appropriate to age.

Wellbeing/Distress (client/carer)

0 Severe/constant: High and constant levels of distress/upset/concern/frustration/anger/embarrassment/withdrawal/severe depression or apathy, unable to express or control emotions appropriately.

1 Frequently severe: Distress/upset/concern/frustration/anger/embarrassment/severe depression/apathy. Becomes concerned easily, requires constant reassurance/support, needs clear/tight limits and structure, loses emotional control easily and/or has difficulty expressing emotions.

2 Moderate consistent: Distress/upset/concern/frustration/anger/embarrassment/withdrawal/severe depression/apathy in unfamiliar situations, frequent emotional encouragement and support required and/or requires encouragement to express emotions.

3 Moderate frequent: Distress/upset/concern/frustration/anger/embarrassment/withdrawal/severe depression/apathy. Controls/expresses emotions with assistance, emotionally dependent on some occasions, vulnerable to change in routine, etc., spontaneously uses methods to assist emotional control.

4 Mild occasional: Distress/upset/concern/frustration/anger/embarrassment/withdrawal/severe depression/apathy. Able to control/express feelings in most situations, generally well adjusted/stable (most of the time/most situations), occasional emotional support/encouragement needed.

5 Not inappropriate: Distress/upset/concern/frustration/anger/embarrassment/withdrawal/severe depression/apathy. Well adjusted, stable and able to cope emotionally with most situations, good insight, accepts and understands own limitations.

2 Augmentative and Alternative Communication (AAC) – Revised

Definition of Augmentative and Alternative Communication

People of all ages with severe speech and language impairments use a range of Augmentative and Alternative Communication (AAC) methods to assist them to communicate their views and needs. AAC is the term used to describe methods of communication which can be added to the more usual methods of speech and writing when these are impaired. AAC can help someone understand as well as express themselves and includes unaided systems such as signing and gesture, and aided systems ranging from pen and paper to the most sophisticated computer technology currently available. Most people who use AAC employ a combination of unaided and aided methods. Aided methods are usually divided into two groups: low-tech and high-tech AAC systems.

NB This scale has been revised since the 3rd edition of the TOM which detailed that it was necessary to consider and score the activity, participation and wellbeing without AAC and with AAC (Enderby & John, 2015, p.102). This has not been found to be practical and it has been decided that clients should be rated in the same way as on other adapted scales, i.e., as they present at a particular time point: initial, intermediate (if required) and at the end of episode of care or discharge.

Identify the descriptor that is 'best fit'. The person rated does not need to have each feature mentioned. Choose the descriptor bearing in mind appropriacy given the age, gender and culture of the individual. Use 0.5 to indicate if patient/client/student is likely to be better or worse than the descriptor. You may choose to give a carer a 'wellbeing' score if that is appropriate to your care plan.

The table below sets out the areas to assess each time a rating is made (i.e., start, interim, final).

Impairment (5 scores)		Activity (1 score)	Participation (1 score)	Wellbeing (1 score)	Carer wellbeing (where relevant)
Physical					
Cognitive					
Sensory					
Speech & Language Output					
Comprehension					

Impairment: Physical

0 Profound abnormality of tone/control/movement, with total body involvement. No voluntary control over any movement.

1 Severe abnormality of tone/control/movement, with total body involvement. Minimal voluntary control of movement.

2 Moderate abnormality of tone/control/movement, with total body involvement or the severe involvement of two limbs. Some reliable movement or gross voluntary control of movement, which may be uncoordinated, very slow or disrupted.

3 Moderate abnormality of tone/control/movement, with partial involvement or severe single limb involvement. Impaired voluntary control of movement, which may be inaccurate and slow.

4 Mild abnormality of tone/control/movement, with mild impairment in voluntary control of movement and control. May have occasional incoordination and inaccuracies.

5 No physical impairment.

Impairment: Cognitive

0 Unresponsive to stimuli.

1 Non-purposeful random and fragmented responses. Occasional response to some simple commands; responses may be severely delayed or inappropriate. Recognizes familiar people and routine tasks in context. Cooperates occasionally. Shows little sign of recall/memory. Can learn simple routines/tasks with maximal assistance.

2 Inconsistent reactions directly related to type of stimulus presented. Occasionally responds appropriately. Response may be delayed but appropriate. Recognizes familiar people in more settings. Can attend but is highly distractible. Unable to focus on individual tasks. Memory may be severely impaired; may perform previously-learned tasks within familiar structure. Insight, judgement and problem-solving are poor.

3 Recognizes familiar people and tasks in most contexts, able to retain small amounts of information consistently. Responds appropriately with some consistency. Appears orientated to setting. Insight, judgement, memory and problem-solving are sometimes unreliable.

4 Alert and able to learn but needs occasional prompting and assistance. Responds well in most situations. Able to recall and integrate past and recent events. Shows carryover for new learning and when activities are learned. Good insight and judgement. May have problems with abstract reasoning in unusual circumstances. Occasional minor memory problem.

5 No cognitive impairment. Good insight, judgement and problem-solving abilities. Responds appropriately. Is alert and able to learn.

Impairment: Sensory – hearing and vision

Rate the person using glasses and hearing aids if normally used.

0 Profound hearing and visual impairment.

1 Severe hearing or visual impairment. Can perceive restricted range of environmental sights or sounds. Limited benefit from hearing aid/glasses.

2 Severe/moderate hearing or visual impairment. Requires attention to perceive a limited range of sights and/or sounds. Benefits from hearing aid/glasses.

3 Moderate hearing or visual impairment. Can hear/see a broad range of environmental sounds and sights. Benefits markedly from hearing aid/glasses.

4 Mild hearing or visual impairment. Occasional difficulty with hearing in some environments or seeing in some lights. Benefits greatly from hearing aid/glasses.

5 No hearing or visual impairment.

Impairment: Speech and language

Output without AAC – you may be helped by reviewing the impairment scales associated with DLD, dysarthria, dysphasia, ASD, etc., as appropriate.

0 Profound presentation of this impairment.

1 Severe presentation of this impairment.

2 Severe/moderate presentation of this impairment.

3 Moderate presentation of this impairment.

4 Mild presentation of this impairment.

5 No impairment.

Impairment: Comprehension

0 Profound difficulty. Comprehension inconsistent even at one keyword level in context.

1 Severe difficulty. Understanding limited to few recognizable words in context or accompanied by visual clues, context, etc.

2 Severe/moderate comprehension difficulty. Can comprehend in familiar context, but inconsistency in ability. Familiar topics of conversation, e.g., familiar names/greetings/basic instructions in context can usually be understood.

3 Moderate comprehension difficulty. Can understand simple sentences and structures, but has difficulty with quick changes of subject, more complex topics or understanding in some contexts when there may be distraction/noise.

4 Mild/occasional difficulty in comprehension. Generally understands most conversation but has difficulty understanding occasionally, e.g., when tired/stressed.

5 No difficulty in comprehending. Normal receptive ability.

Activity: Communication

0 No consistent functional communication. Functioning at pre-intentional level.

1 Limited functional communication. Uses some purposeful responses to indicate limited needs or feelings with informed/familiar communication partners within limited contexts. Can communicate 'yes' and 'no'. Limited communicative intent.

2 Communicates basic needs and information to informed/familiar communication partners. Consistent attempts at purposeful communication in limited contexts. Some communicative intent.

3 Consistent level of communication relating to subjects outside the immediate context. Can transfer more complex messages. Maybe limited in output relating to restricted access to symbol set or other barriers to vocabulary. Some inconsistency. Communicates beyond here and now with familiar persons and in some contexts. Consistent communicative intent.

4 Functional communication available to the individual in most circumstances and with broad range of individuals. Only occasional difficulty. Access to extensive vocabulary which meets needs. May have difficulty/reticence in some environments. Consistent communicative intent.

5 Able to communicate with anyone in any circumstance using broad range of communication modes.

Participation

Autonomy/self-sufficiency/self-reliance = able to determine and have control over one's own viewpoint and not have decisions made by others.

0 Unable to fulfil any social/educational/occupational/recreational/family role. Unable to participate in any situation, even with high-level support. No control over the environment. No social integration.

1 Low self-confidence/poor self-esteem/limited social integration/socially isolated. Unable to fulfil any social/educational/occupational/recreational/or family role. No friends/acquaintances outside family/carers. Only able to engage in social activities with continual support from carers.

2 Some degree of self-sufficiency and social integration beyond immediate family and carers. Fulfilling some social occupational/education/recreational or family role with support. Able to personally effect some decisions/control in familiar situations. Social life is limited and requires involvement of support from carers.

3 Makes decisions and has control over some aspects of life. Able to engage with family/occupation/recreational/education system to some extent with appropriate adjustment and support. Has a few friends/acquaintances. Has some self-sufficiency and control over life. Needs encouragement by others to achieve potential.

4 Can indicate preferences and views in most or all activities. Has broader range of friends. Has only occasional difficulties integrating or in fulfilling social/role activity. May have difficulty in achieving potential in some situations on some occasions. May have restricted interests/pastimes.

5 Can indicate preferences and views in all activities. Able to fulfil social, recreational, occupational educational and family role.

Wellbeing (client/carer)

Do not forget that you can rate the relative or carer on this scale if relevant. Some carers may find that it is more upsetting/frustrating/anxiety-producing when the individual is using technology while others may find the opposite.

0 High and constant levels of distress and problematic emotions, like frustration/elation/anger, etc. May have severe depression and/or severe anxiety. May have severe apathy/social withdrawal. Likely to be unable to express or control emotions appropriately.

1 Severe levels of distress and problematic emotions. These are present all or nearly all of the time. Becomes distressed easily, requires constant reassurance/support, needs clear/tight limits and structure/loses emotional control easily.

2 Moderate-to-severe levels of distress and problematic emotions. Present most of the time. Frequent emotional support required.

3 Moderate levels of distress and problematic emotions which occur frequently. More likely to occur in unfamiliar situations/changes in routine. Controls emotions with assistance, emotionally dependent on some occasions but can use strategies to assist emotional control.

4 Mild levels of distress and problematic emotions. Not present all the time, likely to only be associated with unfamiliar situations or changes of routine. Able to control feelings in most situations, generally well adjusted/stable (most of the time/most situations). Occasional emotional support needed.

5 Not inappropriate. Distress/upset/concern/frustration/anger/embarrassment/withdrawal/severe depression or apathy. Well adjusted, stable and able to cope emotionally with most situations, good insight, accepts and understands own limitations.

3 Autistic Spectrum Disorder

Identify descriptor that is 'best fit'. The patient/client/student does not have to have each feature mentioned. Use 0.5 to indicate if patient/client/student is slightly better or worse than a descriptor and as appropriate to age.

Impairment

0 Profound impairment in multiple areas including verbal communication, nonverbal communication and social interaction. Mute or restricted to a small number of words/phrases/sounds sometimes used repetitively. None or minimal communicative intent. No interest in other people. Reacts negatively to change. Extremely distressed when not in familiar situations or surroundings.

1 Severe/moderate impairment in multiple areas including verbal communication, nonverbal communication, social interaction. Some occasional communicative intent, e.g., making verbal or nonverbal requests to meet some of own needs. Very occasional interest in other people. Mostly reacts negatively to change. Becomes distressed when out of routine.

2 Moderate impairment. May have a reasonable vocabulary but verbal and nonverbal communication deficits will be obvious. Use of language is frequently socially inappropriate, stilted social interaction, limited understanding of social rules. Can tolerate some change in surroundings and routines but needs support/preparation.

3 Moderate/slight impairment. Abnormal or unusual speaking voice and/or manner of speech. Nonverbal communication deficits are obvious to a non-skilled observer, e.g., abnormal posture, no use of hand gestures, limited facial expression. Formulaic social interaction. Difficulty understanding social rules. Can tolerate some changes in surroundings and routines, prefers familiar surroundings and routines.

4 Slight impairment. Difficulties in communication are subtle. May have monotonous voice, pedantic speech or other idiosyncrasies. Rigid thinking style, perhaps evidenced by over-literal interpretations or inability to understand idioms, sarcasm, humour, etc. Social rules are learned but not necessarily natural or automatic. Can manage a range of surroundings and changes in routine.

5 No impairment.

Activity

0 Dependent for all the functional tasks. Unable to meet basic self-care needs. Unable to communicate effectively in any way. Frequently distressed. Repetitive behaviours. Likely to exhibit challenging behaviours.

1 Dependent for most tasks but some cooperation. Able to meet some self-care needs. Limited communication through verbal or nonverbal means which can be interpreted by those familiar with the individual. Very limited understanding of speech, situations and the emotions of others. Likely to have repetitive, purposeless and challenging behaviours.

2 Needs verbal/physical prompts and support/encouragement to initiate/undertake most tasks. Limited understanding of speech, situations and the emotions of others. Able to communicate in a basic way but unable to conduct a flowing conversation. Will be able comprehend obvious nonverbal cues (e.g., can tell if someone is upset if they are crying), but unable to understand more subtle nonverbal cues. May have repetitive, purposeless behaviours in some situations (e.g., hand flapping or other mannerisms). Need for routine, exhibits anxiety/anger in novel situations.

3 Initiates appropriately but might need some support and encouragement to undertake less usual activities. Some understanding of speech, situations and the emotions of others. Able to meet self-care needs. Able to conduct a conversation but it may be stilted or one-sided. Need for routine as above. May have restricted range of interests. May be relatively high functioning in one or two areas. Purposeless, repetitive behaviour absent or less prominent.

4 Able to manage all or nearly all activities of daily living. Some misunderstandings of speech, situations and the emotions of others. Able to communicate effectively with others but has difficulties with subtleties of verbal and nonverbal communication. Social interaction may be less natural, with difficulties appreciating humour, sarcasm, irony. May be seen as 'different' by others, and may be unaware of indiscretions in social situations. A preference for routine. May be exceptionally high functioning in one or two areas.

5 Communicate and functions normally in all situations.

Participation

0 Unable to fulfil any social/occupational/family role. No autonomy. No control and the environment. No social integration.

1 Low self-confidence/poor self-esteem/limited social integration/socially isolated. Unable to fulfil any educational/occupational role. No friends/acquaintances outside family/carers. Only able to engage in social activities with large amounts of support from carers.

2 Some degree of self-confidence and social integration beyond immediate family and carers. Can fulfil some social, occupational, educational, or family role with support. Able to effect some decisions/control in familiar situations. Social life will be very limited.

3 Makes decisions and has control over some aspects of life. Able to engage with family/occupation/recreation/education system to some extent with appropriate adjustment and support. Has a few friends/acquaintances. Has some autonomy and control over life. Needs encouragement to achieve potential.

4 Autonomous in most or all activities. May have occasional difficulties integrating or in fulfilling social/role activity. May have difficulty in achieving potential in some situations on some occasions. May have restricted interests/pastimes.

5 Autonomous in all activities. Able to fill social, occupational and family role.

Wellbeing (client/carer)

0 High and constant levels of distress and problematic emotions, like frustration/elation/anger, etc. May have severe depression and/or severe anxiety. May have severe apathy/social withdrawal. Likely to be unable to express or control emotions appropriately.

1 Severe levels of distress and problematic emotions. These are present all or nearly all of the time. Becomes distressed easily, requires constant reassurance/support, needs clear/tight limits and structure, loses emotional control easily.

2 Moderate-to-severe levels of distress and problematic emotions present most of the time. Frequent emotional support required.

3 Moderate levels of distress and problematic emotions occur frequently, more likely to occur in novel situations/changes in routine. Controls emotions with assistance, emotionally dependent on some occasions, but can use strategies to assist emotional control.

4 Mild levels of distress and problematic emotions. Not present all the time, likely only associated with novel situations or changes of routine. Able to control feelings in most situations, generally well adjusted/stable (most of the time/most situations), occasional emotional support needed.

5 Not inappropriate. Distress/upset/concern/frustration/anger/embarrassment/withdrawal/severe depression or apathy. Well adjusted, stable and able to cope emotionally with most situations, good insight, accepts and understands own limitations.

4 Cardiac Rehabilitation

Identify descriptor that is 'best fit'. The patient/client/student does not have to have each feature mentioned. Use 0.5 to indicate if patient/client/student is slightly better or worse than a descriptor and as appropriate to age.

Impairment

0 Profound. Severe uncontrolled angina, uncontrolled cardiac failure.

1 Some control of cardiac function with multiple drug therapy.

2 Cardiac function and angina mostly controlled with regular medication, at times not controlled.

3 Cardiac function and angina controlled well with regular medication.

4 Cardiac function and angina controlled with occasional or minimal medication.

5 Normal cardiac function.

Activity

0 Lacks functional ability. Totally dependent due to severe chest pain/breathlessness/weakness/dizziness on minimal exertion, i.e., when being transferred bed to chair (room bound).

1 Very limited functional ability. Chest pain/breathlessness/weakness/dizziness limiting activities of daily living, i.e., washing, dressing, mobilizing to toilet (house bound). Constant severe fatigue.

2 Function limited by chest pain/breathlessness/weakness/dizziness, for example, walking on level ground (50 yards) or one flight of stairs (house/immediate environment bound). Becomes fatigued easily.

3 Moderate functional ability. Chest pain/breathlessness/weakness/dizziness on moderate exertion, i.e., one minute each stage of 10-stage exercise circuit (local environment). Periods of fatigue.

4 Mild effect on functional ability. Some occasional reduction in complex or demanding tasks due to pain/breathlessness. Rarely fatigued.

5 No functional disability. Able to tackle normal activities.

Participation

0 Unable to fulfil any social/educational/family role. Not involved in decision making/ no autonomy/no control over environment, no social integration.

1 Low self-confidence/poor self-esteem/limited social integration/socially isolated. Contributes to some basic and limited decisions. Cannot achieve potential in any situation.

2 Some self-confidence/some social integration. Makes some decisions and influences control in familiar situations.

3 Some self-confidence; autonomy emerging. Makes decisions and has control of some aspects of life. Able to achieve some limited social integration/educational activities. Diffident over control over life. Needs encouragement to achieve potential.

4 Mostly confident. Occasional difficulties integrating or in fulfilling social/role activity. Participating in all appropriate decisions. May have difficulty in achieving potential in some situations occasionally.

5 Achieving potential. Autonomous and unrestricted. Able to fulfil social, educational and family role.

Wellbeing/Distress (client/carer)

0 Severe constant: High and constant levels of distress/upset/concern/frustration/anger/ embarrassment/withdrawal/severe depression/apathy, unable to express or control emotions appropriately.

1 Frequently severe: Moderate distress/upset/concern/frustration/anger/embarrassment/ withdrawal/severe depression/apathy. Becomes concerned easily, requires constant reassurance/support, needs clear/tight limits and structure, loses emotional control easily.

2 Moderate consistent: Distress/upset/concern/frustration/anger/embarrassment/ withdrawal/severe depression/apathy in unfamiliar situations. Frequent emotional encouragement and support required.

3 Moderate frequent: Distress/upset/concern/frustration/anger/embarrassment/ withdrawal/severe depression/apathy. Controls emotions with assistance, emotionally dependent on some occasions, vulnerable to change in routine, etc., spontaneously uses methods to assist emotional control.

4 Mild occasional: Distress/upset/concern/frustration/anger/embarrassment/withdrawal/ severe depression/apathy. Able to control feelings in most situations, generally well adjusted/stable (most of the time/most situations), occasional emotional support/ encouragement needed.

5 Not inappropriate: Distress/upset/concern/frustration/anger/embarrassment/withdrawal/ severe depression/apathy. Well adjusted, stable and able to cope emotionally with most situations, good insight, accepts and understands own limitations.

5 Cerebral Palsy

Identify descriptor that is 'best fit'. The patient/client/student does not have to have each feature mentioned. Use 0.5 to indicate if patient/client/student is slightly better or worse than a descriptor and as appropriate to age.

Impairment

0 Profound. Severe abnormality of tone with total body involvement. Fixed or at risk of severe contractures and deformities. No voluntary movement. Severe sensory impairment.

1 Severe abnormality of tone with total body involvement. At risk of severe contractures and deformities. Minimal voluntary movement. Severe sensory impairment.

2 Moderate abnormality of tone with total body involvement or severe involvement of two limbs. At risk of contractures and deformities. Some voluntary movement. Moderate sensory impairment.

3 Moderate abnormality of tone with partial involvement or severe single limb involvement. Little risk of contractures or deformities. Impaired voluntary movement. Mild sensory impairment.

4 Mild abnormality of tone with no contractures and deformities. Mild impairment in voluntary movement. Minimal sensory impairment.

5 No impairment.

Activity

0 No purposeful active movement. Totally dependent on skilled assistance, requires full physical care and constant vigilant supervision. May have totally disruptive and uncooperative behaviour.

1 Some very limited purposeful activity. Bed/chair bound but unable to sit independently. Needs high level of assistance in most tasks. Some awareness, some effort and recognition to contribute to care. Dependent on skilled assistance.

2 Participates in care and engages in some structured activity. Limited self-help skills. Initiates some aspects of activities of daily living (ADL). Transfers with one, mobilizes with two. Requires physical and verbal prompting and supervision for most tasks and movements Dependent on familiar assistant.

3 Appropriately initiates activities. Transfers or walking requires supervision or help of one. Undertakes personal care in modified supported environment. Needs assistance or supervision with some unfamiliar or complex tasks.

4 Carries out personal care and tasks but is less efficient, requires extra time, or may need encouragement, uses prompts effectively. Minimal or occasional assistance required for some complex tasks.

5 Age-appropriate independence.

Participation

0 Unable to fulfil any social/educational/family role. Not involved in decision making/no autonomy/no control over environment; no social integration.

1 Low self-confidence/poor self-esteem/limited social integration/socially isolated. Contributes to some basic and limited decisions. Cannot achieve potential in any situation.

2 Some self-confidence/some social integration/makes some decisions and influences control in familiar situations.

3 Some self-confidence; autonomy emerging. Makes decisions and has control of some aspects of life. Able to achieve some limited social integration/educational activities. Diffident over control over life. Needs encouragement to achieve potential.

4 Mostly confident. Occasional difficulties integrating or in fulfilling social/role activity. Participating in all appropriate decisions. May have difficulty in achieving potential in some situations occasionally.

5 Achieving potential. Autonomous and unrestricted. Able to fulfil social, educational and family role.

Wellbeing/Distress (client/carer)

0 Severe constant: High and constant levels of distress/upset/concern/frustration/anger/embarrassment/withdrawal/severe depression/apathy, unable to express or control emotions appropriately.

1 Frequently severe: Distress/upset/concern/frustration/anger/embarrassment/withdrawal/severe depression/apathy. Becomes concerned easily, requires constant reassurance/support, needs clear/tight limits and structure, loses emotional control easily.

2 Moderate consistent: Distress/upset/concern/frustration/anger/embarrassment/withdrawal/severe depression/apathy in unfamiliar situations, frequent emotional encouragement and support required.

3 Moderate frequent: Distress/upset/concern/frustration/anger/distress/embarrassment/ withdrawal/severe depression/apathy. Controls emotions with assistance, emotionally dependent on some occasions, vulnerable to change in routine, etc., spontaneously uses methods to assist emotional control.

4 Mild occasional: Distress/upset/concern/frustration/anger/embarrassment/withdrawal/ severe depression/apathy. Able to control feelings in most situations, generally well adjusted/stable (most of the time/most situations), occasional emotional support/ encouragement needed.

5 Not inappropriate: Distress/upset/concern/frustration/anger/embarrassment/ withdrawal/severe depression/apathy. Well adjusted, stable and able to cope emotionally with most situations, good insight, accepts and understands own limitations.

6 Developmental Language Disorder (formerly Child Language Impairment)

Identify descriptor that is 'best fit'. The patient/client/student does not have to have each feature mentioned. Use 0.5 to indicate if patient/client/student is slightly better or worse than a descriptor and as appropriate to age.

Impairment

0 Profound language impairment. Profound problems are evident in all areas, extremely limited language involving use, comprehension, expression and phonology.

1 Severe language impairment. Severe problems usually involving all areas, severe problems in two or more areas, one profound overriding area involving use, comprehension, expression and phonology.

2 Severe/moderate language impairment. Severe/moderate problems in some areas. May involve one severe overriding area involving use, comprehension, expression and phonology.

3 Moderate language impairment. Moderate problems in some areas and/or specific moderate problems in one area of language involving use, comprehension, expression, phonology.

4 Mild impairment. Mild problems in one or more areas involving use, comprehension, expression, phonology. Delay sufficient to involve monitoring.

5 No impairment. Age-appropriate language in all areas.

Activity

0 Unable to communicate in any way. No effective understanding even in context.

1 Occasionally able to make basic needs known and able to follow simple instructions in context; can only do this with a trained listener in familiar settings. Minimal communication with maximal assistance.

2 Consistently able to make basic needs known and able to follow simple instructions in context. Communicates better with a trained listener and family members but can occasionally communicate with people that he or she does not know in familiar settings. Depends heavily on context and cues.

3 Consistently able to make needs known but can occasionally convey more information than this. Able to follow most of a conversation in context; can communicate with familiar people or strangers in some unfamiliar as well as familiar settings. Needs some cues and patient/client/student assistance or extra time.

4 Occasional difficulties experienced in effective communication; may have some difficulty with certain people or in specific situations.

5 Communicates well in all situations; age appropriate.

Participation

0 Unable to fulfil any social/educational/family role. Not involved in decision making/ no autonomy/no control over environment, no social integration.

1 Low self-confidence/poor self-esteem/limited social integration/socially isolated. Contributes to some basic and limited decisions. Cannot achieve potential in any situation.

2 Some self-confidence/some social integration/makes some decisions and influences control in familiar situations.

3 Some self-confidence; autonomy emerging. Makes decisions and has control of some aspects of life. Able to achieve some limited social integration/educational activities. Diffident over control over life. Needs encouragement to achieve potential.

4 Mostly confident. Occasional difficulties integrating or in fulfilling social/role activity. Participates in all appropriate decisions. May have difficulty in achieving potential in some situations occasionally.

5 Achieving potential. Autonomous and unrestricted. Able to fulfil social, educational and family role.

Wellbeing/Distress (client/carer)

0 Severe constant: High and constant levels of distress/upset/concern/frustration/ anger/embarrassment/withdrawal/severe depression/apathy. Unable to express or control emotions appropriately.

1 Frequently severe: Moderate distress/upset/concern/frustration/anger/embarrassment/ withdrawal/severe depression/apathy. Becomes concerned easily, requires constant reassurance/support, needs clear/tight limits and structure, loses emotional control easily.

2 Moderate consistent: Distress/upset/concern/frustration/anger/embarrassment/ withdrawal/severe depression/apathy in unfamiliar situations. Frequent emotional encouragement and support required.

3 Moderate frequent: Distress/upset/concern/frustration/anger/embarrassment/ withdrawal/severe depression/apathy. Controls emotions with assistance, emotionally dependent on some occasions, vulnerable to change in routine, etc., spontaneously uses methods to assist emotional control.

4 Mild occasional: Distress/upset/concern/frustration/anger/embarrassment/withdrawal/ severe depression/apathy. Able to control feelings in most situations, generally well adjusted/stable (most of the time/most situations), occasional emotional support/ encouragement needed.

5 Not inappropriate: Distress/upset/concern/frustration/anger/embarrassment/ withdrawal/severe depression/apathy. Well adjusted, stable and able to cope emotionally with most situations, good insight, accepts and understands own limitations.

7 Challenging Behaviour and Forensic Mental Health

Identify the descriptor that is 'best fit'. The patient does not have to have each feature mentioned. Use 0.5 to indicate if patient/client is slightly better or worse than a descriptor and as appropriate to age.

Impairment

0 Profound impairment. Catatonic, unresponsive, no insight, no communicative intent, high levels of hostility, fixed presentation, persistent/severe disturbance of affect, severely emotionally dysregulated. **And/or** daily expression of serious physical aggression/self-injurious behaviour. Regular and frequent use of abusive language. Regular and frequent destruction of significant elements of the environment such as doors, windows, items of furniture. Major legal consequences, e.g., detained under MHA or imprisoned/sentenced to community order/placed on sex offenders' register.

1 Severe thought disorder, variable disturbances of affect, no insight into maladaptive behaviours, some evidence of response, disorientation, severe emotional dysregulation. **And/or** frequent serious physical aggression/self-injurious behaviour. Sustained (several times a week) use of verbal attacks using language which some find offensive. Sustained (several times a week) destruction of significant elements of the environment such as doors, windows, items of furniture. Legal consequences, e.g., fines, antisocial behaviour orders, 'bound over', Guardianship.

2 Severe/moderate thought disorder, disturbance of affect, occasional partial insight, inappropriate responses to some stimuli, severe moderate emotional dysregulation. **And/or** prone to physical aggression/self-injurious behaviour. Frequent use of verbal threats to self or others, and/or offensive language. Frequent (weekly) destruction of significant elements of the environment such as doors, windows, large items of furniture. Significant restrictive or aversive measures are programmed which are subject to procedural regulation and administration.

3 Moderate thought disorder, some insight, some evidence to suggest responsibility of self, some evidence of emotional regulation, signs of orientation, moderate emotional dysregulation. **And/or** occasional physical aggression/self-injurious behaviour when provoked. Occasional (monthly) use of verbal threats to self or others and/or offensive language. Very occasional tendency to destruction of any aspect of the environment.

4 Mild and occasional evidence of some thought disorder, good level of insight, usually stable mood, very occasional disorientation, mild emotional dysregulation and/or very occasional tendency to physical aggression/self-injurious behaviour but uses strategies to modify, very occasional use of aggressive or offensive language. Regulates, mostly successfully, tendency to destroy structures in the environment.

5 No evidence of thought disorder, developed level of insight, orientated, emotionally regulated, clear ability to relate to self and others.

Activity

0 No regards to personal safety or safety of others, may have totally disruptive and uncooperative behaviour. Totally dependent, requires consistent vigilant supervision. Unable to communicate effectively or appropriately in any way. Constant severe challenging behaviour which may include self-harm, assaultive behaviour, self-isolation, verbal aggression, boundary pushing.

1 Minimal regard to personal safety or safety of others. May have some disruptive and/or uncooperative behaviour requiring constant level of assistance and supervision in all tasks. Occasionally able to communicate effectively and appropriately in one context. Minimal communication with maximal assistance. Frequent periods of severe inappropriate, challenging behaviour which may include self-harm, assaultive behaviour, self-isolation, verbal aggression, boundary pushing.

2 Some regard to personal safety or safety of others, cooperative but requires high levels of assistance and supervision in most tasks. Limited functional communication. Consistently able to make basic needs known and able to follow simple instructions out of context. Communicates better with a known communication partner but can occasionally communicate basic needs with unknown people in familiar settings. Depends heavily on context and cues.

3 Requires prompting with regards to maintaining personal safety and safety of others. Needs assistance or supervision with some unfamiliar or complex tasks or in particular contexts. Consistently able to communicate effectively or appropriately in more than one context but not in all situations. Able to follow most simple everyday conversations in context; can communicate just as well with familiar people and strangers in some unfamiliar as well as familiar settings. Needs fewer cues and assistance.

4 Requires advice/support on occasions with regards to maintaining personal safety or safety of others. Needs minimal or occasional assistance required for some complex tasks or new situations. Consistently able to communicate effectively and appropriately in most contexts and often able to communicate in all. Consistently able to convey information but has some difficulty conveying more abstract and complex thoughts. Able to understand almost all everyday conversation but still has occasional difficulty with very complex/lengthy/abstract information. Less context dependent.

5 Independent in all activities. Appropriate engagement with activities.

Participation

0 Unable to fulfil any relationship roles. Not involved in decision making/lacks motivation or responsibility/no investment in self or others/isolates self/lacks trust.

1 Low self-confidence/poor self-esteem. Wary of establishing individual relationships. Unable to take responsibility for self. Seeks to avoid making decisions pertaining to self.

2 Some self-confidence/some social interaction. Able to tolerate some group situations, although does not invest self into these. Still prefers to be alone and defers responsibility for decision making.

3 Some self-confidence/autonomy emerging. More social integration seen through own volition. Beginning to take some decisions with support. Shows more investment in self and willingness to trust others.

4 Mostly confident/occasional difficulties in interaction. Integrating more readily in variety of situations. Shows autonomy when making most decisions. More able to trust a range of people. On occasion does not fulfil relationship potential.

5 Achieving relationship roles/potential/autonomous.

Wellbeing/Distress (client/carer)

0 Severe constant: High and constant levels of distress/upset/concern/frustration/anger/embarrassment/withdrawal/severe depression/apathy. Unable to express or control emotion appropriately.

1 Frequently severe: Moderate distress/upset/concern/frustration/anger/embarrassment/withdrawal/severe depression/apathy. Becomes concerned easily, requires constant reassurance/support, needs clear/tight limits and structure, loses emotional control easily.

2 Moderate consistent: Distress/upset/concern/frustration/anger/embarrassment/withdrawal/severe depression/apathy in unfamiliar situations. Frequent emotional encouragement and support required.

3 Moderate frequent: Distress/upset/concern/frustration/anger/embarrassment/withdrawal/severe depression/apathy. Controls emotions with assistance, emotionally dependent on some occasions, vulnerable to change in routine, etc., spontaneously uses methods to assist emotional control.

4 Mild occasional: Distress/upset/concern/frustration/anger/embarrassment/withdrawal/severe depression/apathy. Able to control feelings in most situations, generally well adjusted/stable (most of the time/most situations), occasional emotional support/encouragement needed.

5 Not inappropriate: Distress/upset/concern/frustration/anger/embarrassment/withdrawal/severe depression/apathy. Well adjusted, stable and able to cope emotionally with most situations, good insight, accepts and understands own limitations.

8 Chronic Pain

Identify descriptor that is 'best fit'. The patient/client/student does not have to have each feature mentioned. Use 0.5 to indicate if patient/client/student is slightly better or worse than a descriptor and as appropriate to age.

Impairment

0 Profound, chronic pain in multiple sites. Severely restricted movement, not relieved by medication or non-pharmacological methods.

1 Constant severe pain in one site, or moderate/frequent intermittent pain in multiple sites. Restricted movement. Little reduction in pain with medication or non-pharmacological methods.

2 Constant moderate pain levels in one site, or pain in multiple sites. Some restriction of movement. Frequent, intermittent relief from medication or other non-pharmacological methods.

3 Moderate/mild pain in one site or pain in multiple sites that occurs intermittently. Occasional improvement from medication or non-pharmacological methods. Minor restriction of movement.

4 Pain that is mostly relieved with medication and/or non-pharmacological methods. Occasional discomfort or restricted movement.

5 No chronic pain.

Activity

0 Bed bound/immobile/totally dependent on for all activities of daily living.

1 Physical assistance needed with most personal activities of daily living.

2 Requires regular assistance with several activities of daily living. Can undertake some tasks independently.

3 Requires minimal assistance and/or supervision and/or adaptions to complete activities of daily living.

4 Independent in familiar and/or adapted environments. Needs occasional assistance and/or extra time with physically demanding activities, due to pain.

5 Activity not restricted by chronic pain.

Participation

0 Unable to fulfil any social, educational or family role. No autonomy. No control over environment. No social integration.

1 Socially isolated/limited social integration. Contact mainly with professionals. No valued family role.

2 Some social integration with assistance. Limited role within one setting.

3 Integrated in a limited number of settings. Needs encouragement or assistance to reach potential. Regularly reduced participation in response to increased pain.

4 Occupies valued roles. Occasional difficulties integrating or in fulfilling social role/ activity when pain increased.

5 Fully integrated, fulfilling a range of valued roles. Not restricted by chronic pain.

Wellbeing/Distress (client/carer)

0 Severe constant: High and constant levels of distress/upset/concern/frustration/ anger/embarrassment/withdrawal/severe depression/apathy. Unable to express or control emotions appropriately.

1 Frequently severe: Moderate distress/upset/concern/frustration/anger/embarrassment/ severe depression/apathy. Becomes concerned easily, requires constant reassurance/ support, needs clear/tight limits and structure, loses emotional control easily and/or has difficulty expressing emotions

2 Moderate consistent: Distress/upset/concern/frustration/anger/embarrassment/ withdrawal/severe depression/apathy in unfamiliar situations, frequent emotional encouragement and support required and/or requires encouragement to express emotions.

3 Moderate frequent: Distress/upset/concern/frustration/anger/embarrassment/ withdrawal/severe depression/apathy. Controls/expresses emotions with assistance, emotionally dependent on some occasions, vulnerable to change in routine, etc., spontaneously uses methods to assist emotional control.

4 Mild occasional: Distress/upset/concern/frustration/anger/embarrassment/withdrawal/ severe depression/apathy. Able to control/express feelings in most situations, generally well adjusted/stable (most of the time/most situations), occasional emotional support/ encouragement needed.

5 Not inappropriate: Distress/upset/concern/frustration/anger/embarrassment/ withdrawal/severe depression/apathy. Well adjusted, stable and able to cope emotionally with most situations, good insight, accepts and understands own limitations.

9 Cleft Lip and Palate

Raters may wish to check whether the Velopharyngeal Dysfunction Scale (in development) is more appropriate for their case. See page 234.

Identify descriptor that is 'best fit'. The patient/client/student does not have to have each feature mentioned. Use 0.5 to indicate if patient/client/student is slightly better or worse than a descriptor and as appropriate to age.

Impairment

0 Profound. Bilateral displaced cleft lip and/or complete cleft palate.

1 Severe. Complete unilateral or bilateral cleft lip and/or cleft palate including more than half of the hard palate.

2 Severe/moderate. Extensive cleft lip and/or cleft palate including more than half of hard palate.

3 Moderate. Moderate lip clefting and/or cleft palate including less than half of hard palate.

4 Mild. Minimal lip clefting and/or cleft palate only of the soft palate. Submucous cleft.

5 Normal lip and palate.

Activity

0 Profound difficulty with speech. Unintelligible. Unable to make recognizable words or sounds. Not understood by familiar or non-familiar listeners. Profound difficulty eating and drinking.

1 Severe problems with articulation. Not intelligible to strangers. Limited to a few recognizable words. Understood by family and friends with help of gestures. Severe problems eating or drinking, much food and all liquids coming down the nose when eating.

2 Severe/moderate problems with articulation. Can produce some single words intelligibly but difficulty with longer utterances. Sounds very hyper/hyponasal. Can usually be understood by friends and family in quiet surroundings but strangers only able to understand occasional words. Severe/moderate difficulty eating and drinking, some food and liquids coming down the nose.

3 Moderate difficulty with articulation, resonance and speech. Speech is different enough to provoke comment. Can be understood by family and friends in most circumstances but understood by non-familiar listeners only when speaking in context. Generally difficult to understand when excited or speaking quickly. Moderate difficulty eating and drinking; no problem with solid food but some liquids come down the nose.

4 Mild difficulty with articulation or resonance and being understood. Understood almost all the time, only occasionally unintelligible when very excited, speaking fast or loudly. Mild problems with nasal regurgitation when drinking.

5 No difficulty in being understood. Normal speech, resonance and feeding for age.

Participation

0 Profound difficulty in participating. Unable to participate in any social/educational/family role. No social integration.

1 Very severe difficulty in participating. Very low opinion of themselves. Very little confidence. Does not mix socially. Never eats or speaks in public. Does not take advantage of any opportunities around them. Will not participate in daily activities like shopping or using the phone.

2 Severe difficulty in participating. Some self-confidence, will mix socially in familiar situations. Avoids mixing and eating with strangers. Needs a lot of support in order to join in. Will accompany friends/family but will not participate in daily activities alone.

3 Moderate difficulty in participating. Reasonably confident. Will mix socially in certain environments. Participates in educational/recreational activities but needs a lot of support and encouragement. Will occasionally make the most of opportunities but seeks assistance with some daily activities like shopping and using the phone.

4 Mild difficulty in participating. Generally self-confident and willing to mix socially in most environments. Participates in family/social/educational decision making. Will make the most of opportunities but occasionally seeks assistance with some daily activities.

5 No difficulty in participating. Fully confident and participates in normal activities appropriate to their age. Well integrated into family/educational/social environment. Will undertake daily activities without assistance

Wellbeing/Distress (client/carer)

0 Profound distress: Constantly severely distressed and embarrassed. Always severely withdrawn, frustrated, apathetic and depressed. Unable to express or control emotions appropriately.

1 Very severe distress: Very frequent episodes of severe distress and embarrassment. Often extremely withdrawn, frustrated, apathetic and depressed in most situations. Needs constant reassurance, encouragement and support. Poor control of emotions.

2 Severe distress: Frequent episodes of distress and embarrassment. Often withdrawn, frustrated, apathetic and depressed in unfamiliar situations. Needs frequent reassurance in unfamiliar situations. Frequent emotional outbursts but generally able to control emotions.

3 Moderate distress: Occasional episodes of distress and embarrassment. Occasionally withdrawn, frustrated, apathetic and depressed in unfamiliar situations. Needs frequent reassurance in unfamiliar environments. Controls emotions with assistance.

4 Mild distress: Generally well adjusted with only a few episodes of distress/ embarrassment/withdrawal/frustration/apathy/depression. Needs occasional reassurance in unfamiliar environments.

5 Not inappropriate: Distress/upset/concern/frustration/anger/embarrassment/ withdrawal/severe depression/apathy.

10 Cognition

Identify descriptor that is 'best fit'. The patient/client/student does not have to have each feature mentioned. Use 0.5 to indicate if patient/client/student is slightly better or worse than a descriptor and as appropriate to age.

Impairment

0 Profound. Unresponsive to all stimuli. Does not recognize people, unable to learn, poor memory responses.

1 Non-purposeful random or fragmented responses. Occasionally responds to some simple commands; may respond to discomfort; responses may be severely delayed or inappropriate. Recognizes some familiar people and routine tasks in context. Cooperates occasionally, attempts to learn simplest routines with maximal assistance.

2 Inconsistent reaction directly related to type of stimulus presented. Occasionally responds appropriately. Can attend but is highly distractible and unable to focus on a particular task. Memory is severely impaired; may perform previously-learned task with structure.

3 Recognizes familiar people and tasks in most contexts, able to retain small amounts of information consistently. Responds appropriately with some consistency, appears oriented to setting, but insight, judgement and problem solving poor. Memory variable – sometimes good, able to cooperate with/learn more complex task.

4 Alert and able to learn but needs occasional prompts and assistance, responds well in most situations. Able to recall and integrate past and recent events; shows carryover for new learning and needs no supervision when activities are learned, but has high-level difficulties, for example abstract reasoning, tolerance for stress, or judgement in unusual circumstances.

5 No cognitive impairment. Responds appropriately, is alert and able to learn.

Activity

0 Inability to recognize body functions and requirements. May have totally disruptive and uncooperative behaviour. Totally dependent, requires full physical care and constant vigilant supervision.

1 Recognizes bodily requirements and occasionally initiates activity but requires a high level of assistance in most tasks.

2 Able to self-care and relate to others in protected environment but is dependent on constant verbal/physical prompting and direction. Skilled assistance required.

3 Needs occasional verbal prompting to initiate activity. Able to operate without supervision for short periods. Able to have some independence with encouragement, independent in familiar surroundings only. General supervision required.

4 Able to live independently with some occasional support, requires extra time, encouragement. Assistance required with unfamiliar tasks.

5 Age-appropriate independence.

Participation

0 Unable to fulfil any social/educational/family role. Not involved in decision making/ no autonomy/no control over environment; no social integration.

1 Low self-confidence/poor self-esteem/limited social integration/socially isolated. Contributes to some basic and limited decisions. Cannot achieve potential in any situation.

2 Some self-confidence/some social integration/makes some decisions and influences control in familiar situations.

3 Some self-confidence; autonomy emerging. Makes decisions and has control of some aspects of life. Able to achieve some limited social integration/educational activities. Diffident over control over life. Needs encouragement to achieve potential.

4 Mostly confident; occasional difficulties integrating or in fulfilling social/role activity. Participates in all appropriate decisions. May occasionally have difficulty in achieving potential in some situations.

5 Achieving potential. Autonomous and unrestricted. Able to fulfil social, educational and family role.

Wellbeing/Distress (client/carer)

0 Severe constant: High and constant levels of distress/upset/concern/frustration/ anger/embarrassment/withdrawal/severe depression/apathy. Unable to express or control emotions appropriately.

1 Frequently severe: Moderate distress/upset/concern/frustration/anger/embarrassment/ withdrawal/severe depression/apathy. Becomes concerned easily, requires constant reassurance/support, needs clear/tight limits and structure, loses emotional control easily.

2 Moderate consistent: Distress/upset/concern/frustration/anger/embarrassment/ withdrawal/severe depression/apathy in unfamiliar situations, frequent emotional encouragement and support required.

3 Moderate frequent: Distress/upset/concern/frustration/anger/embarrassment/ withdrawal/severe depression/apathy. Controls emotions with assistance, emotionally dependent on some occasions, vulnerable to change in routine, etc., spontaneously uses methods to assist emotional control.

4 Mild occasional: Distress/upset/concern/frustration/anger/embarrassment/withdrawal/ severe depression/apathy. Able to control feelings in most situations, generally well adjusted/ stable (most of the time/most situations), occasional emotional support/ encouragement needed.

5 Not inappropriate: Distress/upset/concern/frustration/anger/embarrassment/ withdrawal/severe depression/apathy. Well adjusted, stable and able to cope emotionally with most situations, good insight, accepts and understands own limitations.

11 Complex and Multiple Difficulty

Identify descriptor that is 'best fit'. The patient/client/student does not have to have each feature mentioned. Use 0.5 to indicate if patient/client/student is slightly better or worse than a descriptor and as appropriate to age.

Impairment

0 Profound. No active movement, severe abnormality of muscle tone and patterns of movement. May have abnormal sensory loss, severe fixed deformities, severe respiratory difficulties. Presence of pathological reflexes.

1 Grossly abnormal muscle tone, occasionally some voluntary movement towards stimulus, some contractures, some pathological reflexes, sensory impairment, severely restricted range of movement, frequent respiratory difficulties.

2 Altered muscle tone, some controlled purposeful active movement. Occasional abnormal primitive reflexes. Some joint contractures/fixed limitations, may have sensory impairment.

3 Some useful strength, but abnormal muscle tone, coordinates movement but without accuracy, requires large stable base and low centre of gravity, moderate sensory impairment. Primitive reflexes on pain or noise.

4 Slight abnormality of strength, muscle tone, range of movement; minimal involuntary movements. Slightly impaired neurology with mild weakness or incoordination.

5 Age-appropriate tone, strength, range of movement, coordination and sensation.

Activity

0 No purposeful active movement, totally dependent, requires full physical care and constant vigilant supervision. May have totally disruptive and uncooperative behaviour. Dependent on skilled assistance.

1 Bed/chair bound but unable to sit independently. Some very limited purposeful activity. Needs high level of assistance in most tasks. Some awareness, some effort and recognition to contribute to care. Dependent on skilled assistance.

2 Head and trunk control. Limited self-help skills. Initiates some aspects of ADL. Transfers with one, mobilizes with two. Requires physical and verbal prompting and supervision for most tasks and movements. Participates in care and engaging in some structured activity. Dependent on familiar assistance.

3 Transfers or walking requires supervision or help of one. Undertakes personal care in modified supported environment. Appropriately initiating activities and needs assistance or supervision with some unfamiliar or complex tasks. Initiates activities appropriately.

4 Carries out personal care and tasks but is less efficient, requires extra time or may need encouragement. Uses memory prompts or other aids effectively. Minimal or occasional assistance required for some complex or unfamiliar tasks.

5 Age-appropriate independence.

Participation

0 Unable to fulfil any social/educational/family role. Not involved in decision-making/ no autonomy/no control over environment; no social integration.

1 Low self-confidence/poor self-esteem/limited social integration/socially isolated/ contributes to some basic and limited decisions. Cannot achieve potential in any situation.

2 Some self-confidence/some social integration/makes some decisions and influences control in familiar situations.

3 Some self-confidence; autonomy emerging. Makes decisions and has control of some aspects of life. Able to achieve some limited social integration/educational activities. Diffident over control over life. Needs encouragement to achieve potential.

4 Mostly confident; occasional difficulties integrating or in fulfilling social/role activity. Participates in all appropriate decisions. May occasionally have difficulty in achieving potential in some situations.

5 Achieving potential. Autonomous and unrestricted. Able to fulfil social, educational and family role.

Wellbeing/Distress (client/carer)

0 Severe constant: High and constant levels of distress/upset/concern/frustration/ anger/embarrassment/withdrawal/severe depression/apathy, unable to express or control emotions appropriately.

1 Frequently severe: Moderate distress/upset/concern/frustration/anger/embarrassment/ withdrawal/severe depression/apathy. Becomes concerned easily, requires constant reassurance/support, needs clear/tight limits and structure, loses emotional control easily.

2 Moderate consistent: Distress/upset/concern/frustration/anger/embarrassment/ withdrawal/severe depression/apathy in unfamiliar situations, frequent emotional encouragement and support required.

3 Moderate frequent: Distress/upset/concern/frustration/anger/embarrassment/ withdrawal/severe depression/apathy. Controls emotions with assistance, emotionally dependent on some occasions, vulnerable to change in routine, etc., spontaneously uses methods to assist emotional control.

4 Mild occasional: Distress/upset/concern/frustration/anger/embarrassment/withdrawal/ severe depression/apathy. Able to control feelings in most situations, generally well adjusted/stable (most of the time/most situations), occasional emotional support/ encouragement needed.

5 Not inappropriate: Distress/upset/concern/frustration/anger/embarrassment/ withdrawal/severe depression/apathy. Well adjusted, stable and able to cope emotionally with most situations, good insight, accepts and understands own limitations.

12 Dementia

Identify the descriptor that is 'best fit'. The patient does not have to have each feature mentioned. Use 0.5 to indicate if patient/client is slightly better or worse than a descriptor and as appropriate to age.

Impairment

0 Profound unremitting dementia. Unresponsive to most stimuli. Does not recognize people, unable to attend or concentrate. Severe disorientation, severely impaired short- and long-term memory. Severe and frequent behaviour disturbance. Severely impaired comprehension and expression. No sense of time or place.

1 Severe dementia. Inappropriate, delayed or inconsistent response to stimuli. Occasionally responds to some simple commands associated with the present. Unable to attend to any task. Regular inappropriate behaviour. Occasionally able to communicate basic needs. May use some vocalizations or paralinguistic cues. Marked disorientation significantly impaired short-term memory, impaired long-term memory. Occasionally recognizes familiar people or routine tasks in context.

2 Severe to moderate dementia. Occasionally responds appropriately to stimuli, responds to simple commands, able to understand some simple instructions within context and occasionally expresses appropriately through verbal/nonverbal communication. Occasional behaviour disturbance. Able to recognize relationships in context more consistently. Short-term memory severely impaired. Can attend for short periods but is highly distractible.

3 Moderate dementia. Recognizes familiar people and tasks in most contexts. Able to retain small amounts of information. Short-term memory variable, memory for historical events more intact. Orientated to familiar environments with structure. Very occasional inappropriate behaviour which may be predictable. Able to comprehend everyday conversation within context. Recognizes relationships. Able to express immediate needs but may have word-finding difficulties. Frequently repetitive.

4 Mild dementia. Alert and responds well in most situations. Able to recall most recent events and is orientated in time and place. Able to use strategies in familiar environments but may require repetition or more time to learn. No behaviour disturbance. Able to understand most complex conversation but requires repetition and further explanation. May have some word-finding difficulties and tendency to repeat.

5 No cognitive impairment, responds appropriately, is alert and able to learn.

Activity

0 Inability to recognize and respond appropriately to bodily/biological needs, e.g., thirst/hunger/toileting/pain/temperature, etc. Unable to reliably communicate needs at any time and in any meaningful way. Requires full, skilled assistance to plan, initiate and sustain purposeful activity.

1 Recognizes some bodily/biological needs and occasionally initiates activity but requires a high level of skilled assistance to plan, initiate and sustain purposeful activity. Unable to use strategies, e.g., memory aids. Occasionally may be able to make their needs understood through verbal/nonverbal communication due to familiarity with situation or an individual.

2 Recognizes bodily needs and may initiate activity but requires physical and/or verbal prompting and support to plan, initiate, complete or sustain purposeful activity. Limited functional communication but can occasionally make basic needs understood. Unable to use strategies, e.g., memory aids, without prompting and support. Communicates more consistently with familiar persons. Frequent repetition of instructions required. Meaningful interaction related to here and now.

3 Recognizes and responds appropriately to bodily/biological needs in a familiar environment. Consistently able to make needs known but is inconsistent in less familiar settings. Difficulty using strategies, e.g., memory aids. Needs some verbal prompting to plan/initiate/sustain purposeful activity for tasks. Requires skilled assistance for more complex activities.

4 Able to be independent in routine/familiar tasks, may require occasional verbal prompts/reminders and/or modifications to environment to maintain performance. Can use strategies, e.g., memory aids. Communicates well most of the time and with a wide range of people.

5 Age-appropriate independence.

Participation

0 Unable to fulfil any meaningful and/or purposeful role. Unable to participate in any decision making. No social integration.

1 Requires full, skilled assistance to participate in any purposeful and/or meaningful role. Contributes to some basic and limited decision making. Unable to initiate social integration and socially withdrawn.

2 Some participation in familiar purposeful or meaningful roles. Able to make some basic and limited decisions but unable to predict consequences/outcomes of decisions. Able to engage more readily in some limited social integration. Able to respond to and seek some social integration but will require support to recognize social boundaries.

3 Able to recognize and appropriately participate in purposeful and meaningful roles. Able to make some decisions and understands potential consequences. Able to seek out social integration of their own choice but may not always be socially appropriate.

4 Occasional difficulty in fulfilling purposeful or meaningful roles. Participates in all appropriate decisions. Able to seek out social integration of their choice but may have occasional lapses.

5 Able to fulfil purposeful and meaningful roles. Autonomous decision making and social integration.

Wellbeing/Distress (client/carer)

0 Severe, constant levels of distress: High and constant levels of distress/concern/ anxiety/fear/grief/boredom. Unable to express or control emotions appropriately.

1 Frequently severe levels of distress: Frequent and significant levels of distress/ concern/anxiety/fear/grief/boredom. Infrequent signs of pleasure or enjoyment. Loses emotional control easily.

2 Moderate consistent levels of distress: Signs of distress/concern anxiety/fear/grief/ boredom in unfamiliar situations. Signs of pleasure or enjoyment in familiar situations/ activities. Frequent emotional encouragement and support is required.

3 Moderate frequent levels of distress: Some signs of distress/concern/anxiety/fear/ grief/boredom. Is able to control emotions with assistance but is vulnerable to change in routine. Spontaneously uses methods to assist emotional controls in familiar situations. Frequent signs of pleasure or enjoyment.

4 Mild, occasional levels of distress: Occasional signs of distress/concern/anxiety/fear/ grief/boredom. Able to control feelings in most situations, generally well adjusted/ stable (most of the time/most situations), occasional emotional support/encouragement needed. Frequent and consistent signs of pleasure and enjoyment.

5 Not inappropriate: Distress/upset/concern/frustration/anger/embarrassment/ withdrawal/severe depression/apathy.

13 Diabetes

Identify descriptor that is 'best fit'. The patient/client/student does not have to have each feature mentioned. Use 0.5 to indicate if patient/client/student is slightly better or worse than a descriptor and as appropriate to age.

Impairment

0 Profound. Most severe level of condition. Multiple co-morbidities (e.g., CKD, CVD), modifiable risk factors (e.g., raised BP/lipids/BMI >40 or <16kg/m2) and complex medication regimen which makes weight loss/gain difficult. Severe or regular severe episodes of hypoglycaemia affect activities of daily living, severe symptoms of polyuria, polydypsia. Extremely erratic blood glucose levels, HbA1c >130mmol/l or HbA1c <31mmol/l, blood glucose levels >30mmol/l or <4mmol/l.

1 Severe impairment. Multiple co-morbidities (e.g., CKD, CVD), modifiable risk factors (e.g., raised BP/lipids/BMI >40 or <17kg/m2) requiring multiple medications which make weight loss/gain difficult. Symptoms of polyuria/polydypsia sufficient to have impact on activities of daily living. HbA1c 108-130mmol/mol or HbA1c 31-48 mmol/mol. Erratic blood glucose levels, regular hypoglycaemic episodes alternating with regular hyperglycaemic episodes, blood glucose levels 20-30mmol/l or<4mmol/l.

2 Severe/moderate impairment. One or more co-morbidities (e.g., CKD, CVD)/modifiable risk factors (e.g., raised BP/lipids/ BMI >35 or <18kg/m2) along with medications makes weight loss/gain a challenge. Some symptoms of polyuria, polydypsia/hypoglycaemic episodes which are generally managed and only have slight impact on activities of daily living. HbA1c 75-108 mmol/mol. Unstable blood glucose levels, 12-20mmol/l.

3 Moderate impairment. Associated long-term condition which is well managed. One/two raised modifiable risk factors (e.g., raised BP/lipids BMI >30 or <19kg/m2). Symptoms of polyuria, polydypsia/occasional hypoglycaemic episodes which are not severe and easily self-managed. HbA1c 64-75 mmol/mol, blood glucose levels moderately raised, 11-13mmol/l.

4 Mild impairment. One raised modifiable risk factor. Weight increasing/BMI >25, HbA1c increasing. Increasing requirement for medication. Asymptomatic and manages activities of daily living.

5 No co-morbidities and well controlled modifiable risk factors. BMI 20-25kg/m2 or steady, planned weight reduction. HbA1c to target for individual, stable blood glucose levels.

Activity

0 Bed-bound, totally dependent on others for all care including nutritional needs. Unable to administer own medication or make food choices independently. Dependent on carers to monitor blood glucose levels.

1 House-bound, requiring regular assistance/supervision in activities of daily living. If nutritionally vulnerable may need prompting or some assistance with feeding. Needs help to remember and/or to take medication appropriately. Needs support from carers to check blood glucose levels.

2 Moderate limitations, needs prompting/encouragement from carers to eat regularly, modify diet, check blood glucose levels and to take medication correctly.

3 Moderate limitations on ability, may need some support from others or extra time/investment/support in knowledge, confidence, skills, attitude, and motivation around food choices/meal planning/self-administration of medication. Needs support to self-care and self-monitor blood glucose levels.

4 Mild limitations on ability to self-manage, may need occasional support or prompting, e.g., to take medication appropriately and monitor blood glucose levels or to access appropriate diet.

5 Completely independent, able to exercise at a level appropriate for age, able to self-manage without support. Accesses appropriate diet, able to self-adjust own insulin and knows when to access support if medication needs review. Self-monitors blood glucose appropriately and acts on information obtained to maintain excellent diabetes control.

Participation

0 No autonomy, isolated, no social family role.

1 Very limited choices, contact mainly with professionals, no social or family role, little control over life, limited ability to make lifestyle choices, food choices, treatment options.

2 Some integration, value and autonomy in one setting.

3 Integrated, valued and in autonomy in limited number of settings.

4 Occasionally some restriction in autonomy, integration or role. Can do things independently but has some barriers.

5 Integrated, valued, occupies appropriate role, takes responsibility for own health.

Wellbeing/Distress (client/carer)

0 Severe constant: High and constant levels of distress/upset/concern/frustration/anger/embarrassment/withdrawal/severe depression/apathy, unable to express or control emotions appropriately.

1 Frequently severe: Moderate distress/upset/concern/frustration/anger/embarrassment/withdrawal/severe depression/apathy. Becomes concerned easily, requires constant reassurance/support, needs clear/tight limits and structure, and loses emotional control easily.

2 Moderate consistent: Distress/upset/concern/frustration/anger/embarrassment/withdrawal/severe depression/apathy in unfamiliar situations, frequent emotional encouragement and support required.

3 Moderate frequent: Distress/upset/concern/frustration/anger/embarrassment/withdrawal/severe depression/apathy. Controls emotions with assistance, emotionally dependent on some occasions, vulnerable to change in routine, etc., spontaneously uses methods to assist emotional control.

4 Mild occasional: Distress/upset/concern/frustration/anger/embarrassment/withdrawal/severe depression/apathy. Able to control feelings in most situations, generally well adjusted/stable (most of the time/most situations), occasional emotional support/encouragement needed

5 Not inappropriate (behaves appropriately in situation): Distress/upset/concern/frustration/anger/embarrassment/withdrawal/severe depression/apathy. Well adjusted, stable and able to cope emotionally with most situations, good insight, accepts and understands own limitations.

14 Dietetic Intervention for the Prevention of Cardiovascular Disease

Post event, e.g., heart attack; stroke.
   Identify descriptor that is best fit. The patient/client/student does not have to have each feature mentioned. Use 0.5 to indicate if patient/client/student is slightly better or worse than a descriptor and as appropriate to age.

Impairment

0 Multiple co-morbidities including other vascular disease, e.g., diabetes, CKD, vascular dementia, previous stroke/MI. Complex medication regimen. All modifiable risk factors present: raised lipids, raised BP and outside healthy weight range.

1 More than one co-morbidity including other vascular disease, e.g., diabetes, CKD, vascular dementia, previous stroke/MI. Requires multiple medications and has a number of modifiable risk factors, e.g., raised lipids, BP, BMI outside healthy range.

2 Has one other co-morbidity, e.g., diabetes, requires a number of medications and has more than one modifiable risk factor, e.g., raised lipids, BP, BMI outside healthy range.

3 Has one other co-morbidity and one raised modifiable risk factor, e.g., raised lipids, BP, BMI outside healthy range.

4 No co-morbidities, limited number of medications required, one raised modifiable risk factor, e.g., raised lipids, BP, BMI outside healthy range.

5 Healthy weight, no co-morbidities. No modifiable risk factors. No other vascular conditions.

Activity

0 Totally dependent on others (carers and staff) for nutritional needs, e.g., shopping, cooking and assisted feeding. Nutrition support indicated. Very severe cognition, communication and limited ability to support nutrition.

1 Severe limitations, requires regular assistance, supervision from carers, staff to follow a cardio-protective diet or, if nutritionally vulnerable, meets requirements through oral nutritional support/partially dependent on others to access food.

2 Moderate limitations, e.g., needs prompting from carers to follow a cardio-protective diet or, if nutritionally vulnerable, meets requirements through oral nutritional support on a temporary basis, some access issues around food.

3 Moderate-to-mild limitations on ability to follow a cardio-protective diet, e.g., needs extra time, investment in knowledge, confidence, skills, attitude around shopping, cooking and meal planning or might need some prompting.

4 Mild limitations on ability to follow a cardio-protective diet, e.g., needs first line advice, resources to increase knowledge, confidence, skills, and attitudes around shopping, cooking and meal planning. No issues with access to food.

5 Completely independent and able to follow a cardio-protective diet and access food independently.

Participation

0 No autonomy, isolated, no social family role.

1 Very limited choices, contact mainly with professionals, no social or family role, little control over life, limited ability to make lifestyle choices, food choices, treatment options.

2 Some integration, value and autonomy in one setting.

3 Integrated, valued and in autonomy in limited number of settings.

4 Occasionally some restriction in autonomy, integration or role, can do things independently but has some barriers.

5 Integrated, valued, occupies appropriate role, takes responsibility for own health.

Wellbeing/Distress (client/carer)

0 Severe constant: High and constant levels of distress/upset/concern/frustration/ anger/embarrassment/withdrawal/severe depression/apathy, unable to express or control emotions appropriately.

1 Frequently severe: Moderate distress/upset/concern/frustration/anger/embarrassment/ withdrawal/severe depression/apathy. Becomes concerned easily, requires constant reassurance, support, needs clear, tight limits and structure and loses emotional control easily.

2 Moderate consistent: Distress/upset/concern/frustration/anger/embarrassment/ withdrawal/severe depression/apathy in unfamiliar situations, frequent emotional encouragement and support required.

3 Moderate frequent: Distress/upset/concern/frustration/anger/embarrassment/ withdrawal/severe depression/apathy. Controls emotions with assistance, emotionally dependent on some occasions, vulnerable to change in routine, etc., spontaneously uses methods to assist emotional control

4 Mild occasional: Distress/upset/concern/frustration/anger/embarrassment/withdrawal/ severe depression/apathy. Able to control feelings in most situations, generally well adjusted, stable (most of the time, most situations), occasional emotional support, encouragement needed.

5 Not inappropriate (behaves appropriately in situation): Distress/upset/concern/ frustration/anger/embarrassment/withdrawal/severe depression/apathy. Well adjusted, stable and able to cope emotionally with most situations, good insight, accepts and understands own limitations.

15 Dietetic Intervention for Enteral Feeding: Paediatrics*

*Reliability requires further testing.

Identify descriptor that is 'best fit'. The patient/client/student does not have to have each feature mentioned. Use 0.5 to indicate if patient/client/student is slightly better or worse than a descriptor and as appropriate to age.

Impairment

0 Nutritionally unstable. Persistent growth faltering or severe, constant enteral feeding-associated symptoms that remain unresolved by frequent, unplanned interventions and are not attributable to disease progression.

1 Nutritionally unstable. Persistent growth faltering or severe, regular enteral feeding-associated symptoms resolved by frequent, unplanned interventions and not attributable to disease progression.

2 Nutritionally unstable or has severe, occasional enteral feeding-associated symptoms that are not attributable to disease progression and are resolved by frequent, planned interventions.

3 Nutritional needs are changing as a result of disease progression, etc., or moderate, occasional enteral feeding-associated symptoms resolved by frequent, planned interventions to revise feeding regimen. Nutritional goals are achieved.

4 Working towards achieving nutritional/other goals (e.g., achieving expected growth and tolerance), rarely has enteral feeding-associated symptoms requiring planned, routine intervention to review stoma site and/or nutrition/hydration status, etc.

5 Nutritional goals are met/no enteral feeding-associated symptoms. Requires planned, routine intervention to monitor stoma site and/or nutrition/hydration status, etc.

Activity

0 Parent/child is totally dependent on others for care related to enteral feeding/nutrition. Care package is provided by external agency/community nursing. Frequent respite care required.

1 Parent/child is totally dependent on others. Care regarding enteral feeding/nutrition is provided by external care agencies/community nursing and by family living with patient. Frequent respite care required.

2 Parent/child is totally dependent on others and supported by external agencies/ community nursing.

3 Parent/child is partially dependent for care related to enteral feeding/nutrition. Parent/child requires some assistance with enteral feeding from community nursing.

4 Parent/child is partially dependent for care related to enteral feeding/nutrition. Patient requires some assistance with enteral feeding/nutrition from community nursing.

5 Parent/child is completely independent with own care around enteral feeding/nutrition. requiring little support from community nursing and healthcare professionals.

Participation

0 Carer/child has no autonomy, isolated, no social family role and lifestyle determined by medical condition and feeding.

1 Carer/child has very limited choices, contact mainly with professionals, no social or family role, little control over life, and lifestyle largely determined by medical condition and feeding.

2 Carer/child has some integration, value and autonomy in one setting.

3 Carer/child is integrated, valued and has autonomy in limited number of settings.

4 Carer/child occasionally has some restriction in autonomy integration or role, can do things independently but has some barriers.

5 Carer/child is integrated, valued, occupies appropriate role, takes responsibility for own health and able to participate in age-appropriate activities.

Wellbeing/Distress (client/carer)

0 Severe constant: High and constant levels of distress/upset/concern/frustration/ anger/embarrassment/withdrawal/severe depression/apathy, unable to express or control emotions appropriately.

1 Frequently severe: Moderate distress/upset/concern/frustration/anger/embarrassment/ withdrawal/severe depression/ apathy. Becomes concerned easily, requires constant reassurance/support, needs clear/tight limits and structure, and loses emotional control easily.

2 Moderate consistent: Distress/upset/concern/frustration/anger/embarrassment/ withdrawal; severe depression/apathy in unfamiliar situations, frequent emotional encouragement and support required.

3 Moderate frequent: Distress/upset/concern/frustration/anger/embarrassment/withdrawal/severe depression/apathy. Controls emotions with assistance, emotionally dependent on some occasions, vulnerable to change in routine, etc., spontaneously uses methods to assist emotional control.

4 Mild occasional: Distress/upset/concern/frustration/anger/embarrassment/withdrawal/severe depression/apathy. Able to control feelings in most situations, generally well adjusted/stable (most of the time/most situations), occasional emotional support/encouragement needed.

5 Not inappropriate (behaves appropriately in situation): Distress/upset/concern/frustration/anger/embarrassment/withdrawal/severe depression/apathy. Well adjusted, stable and able to cope emotionally with most situations, good insight, accepts and understands own limitations.

16 Dietetic Intervention for Home Enteral Feeding: Adult[*]

*Reliability is requiring further testing.

Identify descriptor that is 'best fit'. The patient/client does not have to have each feature mentioned. Use 0.5 to indicate if patient/client is slightly better or worse than a descriptor and as appropriate to age.

Impairment

0 Profound nutritional instability (e.g., >10% weight loss in 3-6 months) or severe, constant enteral feeding-associated symptoms that remain unresolved by frequent, unplanned interventions.

1 Severe nutritional instability (e.g., significant unintentional weight loss) or severe, regular enteral feeding-associated symptoms resolved by frequent, unplanned ('crisis') interventions. Nutritional goals hard to achieve.

2 Severe/moderate nutritional instability or severe but not regular enteral feeding-associated symptoms managed by frequent, planned interventions. Improvement towards nutritional goals.

3 Moderate predictable nutritional needs or moderate and occasional enteral feeding-associated symptoms managed by frequent, planned interventions to revise feeding plan. Nutritional goals are achieved.

4 Working towards achieving nutritional/other goals (e.g., weight, wound healing, patient is more alert), rarely has enteral feeding-associated symptoms. Requires planned routine professional follow-up to review, e.g., stoma site and/or nutrition/hydration status, etc.

5 Nutritional/other goals are met and stable, no enteral feeding-associated symptoms.

Activity

0 Totally dependent on others for care related to enteral feeding/nutrition and activities of daily living.

1 Totally dependent on others but can participate in activities of daily living and care relating to enteral feeding/nutrition.

2 Can initiate and assist with activities of daily living and carer relating to enteral feeding/nutrition. Care regarding enteral feeding/nutrition is provided by nonprofessionals/carers/family members.

3 Partially dependent for care related to activities of daily living and enteral feeding/nutrition. Patient requires some assistance with enteral feeding/nutrition from others. May need encouragement and support.

4 Occasionally requires assistance/advice/support for certain activities of daily living or aspects of enteral feeding/nutrition.

5 Completely independent with own care.

Participation

0 No autonomy, isolated, no social family role.

1 Very limited choices, contact mainly with professionals, no social or family role, little control over life, limited ability to make lifestyle choices, food choices, treatment options.

2 Some integration, value and autonomy in one setting.

3 Integrated, valued and in autonomy in limited number of settings.

4 Occasionally some restriction in autonomy, integration or role, can do things independently but has some barriers.

5 Integrated, valued, occupies appropriate role, takes responsibility for own health.

Wellbeing/Distress (client/carer)

0 Severe constant: High and constant levels of distress/upset/concern/frustration/anger/embarrassment/withdrawal/severe depression/apathy, unable to express or control emotions appropriately.

1 Frequently severe: Moderate distress/upset/concern/frustration/anger/embarrassment/withdrawal/severe depression/apathy. Becomes concerned easily, requires constant reassurance/support, needs clear/tight limits and structure, and loses emotional control easily.

2 Moderate consistent: Distress/upset/concern/frustration/anger/embarrassment/withdrawal/severe depression/apathy in unfamiliar situations, frequent emotional encouragement and support required.

3 Moderate frequent: Distress/upset/concern/frustration/anger/embarrassment/withdrawal/severe depression/apathy. Controls emotions with assistance, emotionally dependent on some occasions, vulnerable to change in routine, etc., spontaneously uses methods to assist emotional control.

4 Mild occasional: Distress/upset/concern/frustration/anger/embarrassment/withdrawal/ severe depression/apathy. Able to control feelings in most situations, generally well adjusted/stable (most of the time/most situations), occasional emotional support/ encouragement needed.

5 Not inappropriate (behaves appropriately in situation): Distress/upset/concern/ frustration/anger/embarrassment/withdrawal/severe depression/apathy. Well adjusted, stable and able to cope emotionally with most situations, good insight, accepts and understands own limitations.

17 Dietetic Intervention for Irritable Bowel Syndrome

Identify descriptor that is 'best fit'. The patient/client/student does not have to have each feature mentioned. Use 0.5 to indicate if patient/client/student is slightly better or worse than a descriptor and as appropriate to age.

Impairment

0 Profound. Most severe level of condition, e.g., IBS with diarrhoea, enduring severe pain, bloating, constipation, urgency, bleeding persistently. On multiple medications/interventions, specific for IBS. Continual symptoms no relief.

1 Severe condition, e.g., IBS with diarrhoea, severe pain, bloating, constipation, urgency daily. On several medications/interventions specific for IBS. Very frequent symptoms.

2 Severe, moderate condition, e.g., IBS with diarrhoea, pain, bloating, constipation, distress, urgency daily. On limited medications/interventions specific for IBS. Frequent symptoms.

3 Moderate condition, e.g., IBS with diarrhoea, discomfort, bloating, constipation, urgency several times a week. On medication/intervention specific for IBS as required. Symptoms can be stabilized with the use of one/two interventions.

4 Mild condition, e.g., IBS with diarrhoea, mild discomfort, bloating, constipation, urgency. On no medication/intervention specific for IBS. Symptoms can stabilize spontaneously and/or with simple lifestyle changes. Very occasional symptoms.

5 No condition or recent symptoms of condition within the last 3–6 months.

Activity

0 Hospitalized due to severity of symptoms.

1 House-bound due to severity of symptoms.

2 Severe restrictions on leaving home and activities; can leave house with assistance from others and undertake short-lived/infrequent activities.

3 Impaired ability to undertake normal activities/leave house/work/school independently occasionally when symptoms dictate.

4 Infrequent/occasional limitations on activity.

5 No limitations on normal activity. Completely independent.

Participation

0 No autonomy; isolated, no family/social role.

1 Very limited choices, contact mainly with professionals, no social or family roles, little control over life.

2 Some integration, value and autonomy in one setting.

3 Integrated, valued and autonomous in limited number of settings.

4 Occasionally some restriction on autonomy, integration or role.

5 Integrated, valued, occupies appropriate role.

Wellbeing/Distress (client/carer)

0 Severe constant: High and constant levels of distress/upset/concern/frustration/anger/embarrassment/withdrawal/severe depression/apathy. Unable to express or control emotions appropriately (unable to cope), e.g., constant anxiety around continence; or anxiety/concern around allergens which dominates their life.

1 Frequently severe: Moderate levels of distress/upset/concern/frustration/anger/embarrassment/withdrawal/severe depression/apathy. Becomes concerned easily, requires constant reassurance/support, needs clear/tight limits and structure, loses emotional control easily, e.g., struggles to relax as frequently distressed/concerned, etc., regarding continence, allergens.

2 Moderate consistent: Distress/upset/concern/frustration/anger/embarrassment/withdrawal/severe depression/apathy in unfamiliar situations. Frequent emotional encouragement and support required, e.g., does not know where the next toilet is or apprehensive about making menu choices when eating out.

3 Moderate frequent: Distress/upset/concern/frustration/anger/embarrassment/withdrawal/severe depression/apathy. Controls emotions with assistance, emotionally dependent on some occasions, vulnerable to change in routine, etc., spontaneously uses methods to assist emotional control, e.g., plans toilet route and phones restaurant ahead of time.

4 Mild occasional: Distress/upset/concern/frustration/anger/embarrassment/withdrawal/severe depression/apathy. Able to control feelings in most situations, generally well adjusted/stable (most of the time/most situations), occasional emotional encouragement and support needed. Copes well with most situations, develops coping strategies, e.g., rarely needs to phone relatives/a friend for emotional support if a distressing situation occurs.

5 Not inappropriate (behaves appropriately in situation): Distress/upset/concern/frustration/anger/embarrassment/withdrawal/severe depression/apathy. Well adjusted, stable and able to cope emotionally with most situations, good insight, accepts and understands own limitations. Has coping strategies for most situations.

18 Dietetic Intervention for Obesity: Paediatric

Identify descriptor that is 'best fit'. The patient/client/student does not have to have each feature mentioned. Use 0.5 to indicate if patient/client/student is slightly better or worse than a descriptor and as appropriate to age.

Impairment

0 BMI >4 standard deviations above 50th centile. Presence of several co-morbidities, e.g., respiratory problems, tissue viability issues, sleep apnoea, fatty liver, and limiting effect on mobility/development.

1 BMI >3.5 standard deviations above 50th centile. One or multiple chronic co-morbidities, e.g., respiratory problems, tissue viability issues, sleep apnoea, fatty liver, and limiting effect on mobility/development.

2 BMI >2.67 standard deviations above 50th centile. Mobility/development may be affected and there may be some presence/elevated cholesterol levels or blood pressure.

3 BMI >98th centile. Mobility/development may be affected and there may be some presence/elevated cholesterol levels or blood pressure.

4 BMI >91st centile. Overweight. Weight of increasing risk to health. Free from associated conditions.

5 Within healthy weight range.

Activity

0 Carer/child is totally dependent on others for nutritional needs, e.g., shopping, cooking, self-care.

1 Carer/child requires regular assistance/supervision from carers/staff to self-care, make dietary and other lifestyle choice, partially dependent on others to access food or to be physically active.

2 Carer/child has moderate limitations, e.g., needs prompting from carers to follow a weight management care plan, some access issues around food.

3 Carer/child has mild limitations on ability to follow a weight management care plan, e.g., needs extra time/investment/support in knowledge, confidence, skills, attitude/motivation around food choice, cooking and meal planning, needs support to self-care and self-monitor.

4 Carer/child has mild limitations on ability to follow a weight management care plan, e.g., needs first line advice/resources to increase knowledge, confidence, skills, attitudes/motivation around food choice, cooking and meal planning. No issues with access to food.

5 Carer/child is completely independent, able and motivated to follow a weight management care plan, makes informed independent food and activity choices and able to self-monitor.

Participation

0 Carer/child has no autonomy/is isolated, no family/social role, little or no choice over what is eaten/provided.

1 Carer/child shows very limited food choice, contact mainly with professionals, no social or family roles, little control over life what is eaten, i.e., eats what is provided/apathy related to food or support to be physically active.

2 Carer/child has some integration, value and autonomy in one setting due to lack of support/environment, routinely struggles to implement dietary changes.

3 Carer/child is integrated, valued and autonomous in limited number of settings due to lack of support/environment, struggles sometimes to implement dietary changes.

4 Carer/child occasionally has some restriction on autonomy, integration or role, can't always make healthy choices (environment vs personal responsibility).

5 Integrated, valued, good role model for others in eating a healthy diet.

Wellbeing/Distress (client/carer)

0 Severe constant: Carer/child shows high and constant levels of distress/upset/concern/frustration/anger/embarrassment/guilt/shame/withdrawal/severe depression/apathy regarding weight, shape and eating. Unable to express or control emotions appropriately. Eating behaviours strongly linked to wellbeing, strong sense of lack of control with eating, eating and food used as a coping strategy for other emotions.

1 Frequently severe: Carer/child shows moderate levels of distress/upset/concern/frustration/anger/embarrassment/guilt/shame withdrawal/severe depression apathy. Becomes concerned easily, requires constant reassurance/support, needs clear/tight limits and structure, loses emotional control easily, low mood. Strong sense of lack of control with eating. Eating behaviours strongly linked to wellbeing, eating and food used as a coping strategy for other emotions.

2 Carer/child feels anxious/depressed about future health or lacks insight/denial. Black and white thinking about eating behaviours, anxiety about body shape, often feels lacks control with eating behaviours/food, frequently uses food and eating as a coping strategy for other emotion/guilt/shame. Feels emotions of guilt and shame. Needs reassurance and support.

3 Carer/child occasionally feels anxious about shape and weight, has some black and white thoughts and beliefs about food and weight. Realistic view of ability to implement changes and weight loss goals.

4 Carer/child feels mildly concerned about their future health. Able to implement changes to eating behaviour, does not relate food to controlling emotional wellbeing.

5 Not inappropriate: Distress/upset/concern/frustration/anger/embarrassment/withdrawal/severe depression/apathy.

19 Dietetic Intervention for Obesity: Adult

Identify descriptor that is 'best fit'. The patient/client/student does not have to have each feature mentioned. Use 0.5 to indicate if patient/client/student is slightly better or worse than a descriptor and as appropriate to age.

Impairment

0 Profound level of obesity, BMI >40kg/m. Several severe co-morbidities involving cardiac and respiratory systems, pressure sores. Physiological effects such that there is no exercise tolerance. Associated health conditions and medications may make weight loss difficult.

1 Severe obesity. One severe or multiple less severe co-morbidities, e.g., cardiac, respiratory problems, tissue viability issues, diabetes, sleep apnoea, fatty liver. Associated health conditions and medications may make weight loss difficult.

2 Severe/moderate obesity. Moderate co-morbidities, e.g., osteoarthritis, diabetes, sleep apnoea, high blood pressure, fatty liver. Associated health conditions and medications may make weight loss difficult.

3 Moderate obesity. Some associated conditions and physiological effects: osteoarthritis, controlled diabetes, weakness and reduced muscle power.

4 Overweight. Weight increasing risk to health, mild physiological effects. Mildly reduced exercise tolerance.

5 No obesity, BMI 25, within healthy weight range. Age-appropriate exercise tolerance.

Activity

0 Bedbound, unable to alter position. Totally dependent on others for all physical/ nutritional care needs. Very severe constant shortness of breath on any attempt to move. Physiological effects such that there is no exercise tolerance.

1 Severe limitations, requires regular assistance/supervision from carers/staff to self-care. Able to assist with some basic tasks of daily living, i.e., eating, washing upper body. Severe shortness of breath with activity. Physiological effects such that there is severely limited exercise tolerance.

2 Walks or self-propels over short distances, i.e., on level ground (50 metres). Physiological effects such that there is very restricted exercise tolerance. Able to undertake gentle exercise or daily living tasks for maximum of 10 minutes before experiencing shortness of breath.

3 Walks or self-propels around local environment. Participates in gentle exercise for 20 minutes or moderate exercise for 10 minutes before experiencing shortness of breath. Mild limitations on ability to follow a weight management care plan, e.g., needs extra time/support in knowledge, skills, attitude/motivation around food choice, cooking and meal planning, needs support to self-care and self-monitor.

4 Walks or self-propels over long distances. Participates in moderate exercise or daily living tasks for 20 minutes or cardiorespiratory exercise for 10 minutes before experiencing shortness of breath. Mild limitation of ability to follow a weight management care plan, e.g., needs first line advice/resources to increase knowledge, skills, attitude/motivation around food choice, cooking and meal planning.

5 Completely independent. Participates in full exercise regime appropriate to age. Able and motivated to follow a weight management care plan, makes informed independent food and activity choices and able to self- monitor.

Participation

0 No autonomy, isolated, no social family role.

1 Very limited choices, contact mainly with professionals, no social or family role, little control over life, limited ability to make lifestyle choices, food choices, and treatment options.

2 Some integration, value and autonomy in one setting.

3 Integrated, valued and in autonomy in limited number of settings.

4 Occasionally some restriction in autonomy, integration or role, can do things independently but has some barriers.

5 Integrated, valued, occupies appropriate role, takes responsibility for own health.

Wellbeing/Distress (client/carer)

0 Severe constant: High and constant levels of distress/upset/concern/frustration/ anger/embarrassment/guilt/shame/withdrawal/severe depression/apathy regarding weight, shape and eating. Unable to express or control emotions appropriately. Eating behaviours strongly linked to wellbeing, strong sense of lack of control with eating. Eating and food used as a coping strategy for other emotions.

1 Frequently severe: Severe/moderate levels of distress/upset/concern/frustration/anger/embarrassment/guilt/shame/withdrawal/severe depression/apathy. Becomes concerned easily, requires constant reassurance/support, needs clear/tight limits and structure, loses emotional control easily, low mood. Strong sense of lack of control with eating. Eating behaviours strongly linked to wellbeing. Eating and food used as a coping strategy for other emotions.

2 Moderate levels of distress/upset/concern/frustration/anger/embarrassment/guilt/shame/withdrawal/severe depression/apathy. Feels anxious/depressed about future health or lacks insight/denial. Black and white thinking about eating behaviours, anxiety about body shape, often feels lacks control with eating behaviours, food. Frequently uses food and eating as a coping strategy for other emotions, e.g., guilt/shame. Needs reassurance and support.

3 Moderate/mild levels of distress/upset/concern/frustration/anger/embarrassment/guilt/shame/withdrawal/severe depression/apathy. Occasionally feels anxious about shape and weight, has some black and white thoughts and beliefs about food and weight. Realistic view of ability to implement changes and weight loss goals.

4 Mild levels of distress/upset/concern/frustration/anger/embarrassment/guilt/shame/withdrawal/severe depression/apathy. Feels mildly concerned about their future health. Able to implement changes to eating behaviour, does not relate food to controlling emotional wellbeing.

5 Not inappropriate: Distress/upset/concern/frustration/anger/embarrassment/withdrawal/severe depression/apathy.

20 Dietetic Intervention for Undernutrition: Paediatrics

Identify descriptor that is 'best fit'. The patient/client/student does not have to have each feature mentioned. Use 0.5 to indicate if patient/client/student is slightly better or worse than a descriptor and as appropriate to age.

Impairment

0 More than 3 centiles between plotted weight and length/height, head circumference, length/height faltering, impact on developmental milestones. Specific nutritional deficiencies. Severe deficit in meeting estimated nutritional requirements.

1 More than 3 centiles between plotted weight and length/height, negative impact on developmental milestones. Some specific nutritional deficiency. Significant deficit in meeting estimated nutritional requirements.

2 More than 2 centiles between weight and length/height and specific nutritional deficiency or more than 3 centiles between weight and length/height.

3 More than 2 centiles between weight and length/height. May be meeting nutritional requirements.

4 Progressing/making acceptable growth across centiles, improvement in developmental milestones.

5 No recent unintentional weight loss or faltering. Currently meeting nutritional needs.

Activity

0 Child requires full assistance for eating or drinking. No appetite. No willingness to eat. Severe food refusal or barriers to feeding.

1 Child needs a considerable amount of assistance to eat and drink. Very reduced appetite. Mostly unwilling to eat. Significant food refusal or barriers to eating/feeding.

2 Child may need some assistance when eating or drinking. Reduced appetite. Frequently unwilling to eat. Some food refusal or barriers to eating/feeding.

3 Child/carer requires some support such as prompting or adaptations for eating/feeding. Variable appetite. Occasionally unwilling to eat/feed. Occasional food refusal or barriers to eating/feeding.

4 Able to feed appropriately for age, may require some adaptations or encouragement. Occasional suppressed appetite. Willing to eat/feed.

5 Able to eat and drink appropriately for age. Has a full appetite. Willing to eat/feed.

Participation

0 Child is isolated, no social family role at mealtimes, withdrawn, refusal.

1 No social or family role at mealtimes, no engagement in choices offered, refusal.

2 Some integration in one setting, limited acceptance of nutrition, refusal.

3 Integrated in limited number of settings, acceptance of increasing quantity of nutrition.

4 Integrated in most settings and participates in social role of eating/feeding, may still be some barriers to eating/feeding.

5 No refusal of nutrition and integrates and engages appropriately at feed/mealtimes.

Wellbeing/Distress (client/carer)

0 Severe constant: Child/carer experiences high and constant levels of distress/upset/ concern/frustration/anger/embarrassment/withdrawal/severe depression/apathy, unable to express or control emotions appropriately.

1 Frequently severe: Child/carer experiences moderate distress/upset/concern/ frustration/anger/embarrassment/withdrawal/severe depression/apathy. Becomes concerned easily, requires constant reassurance/support, needs clear/tight limits and structure and loses emotional control easily.

2 Moderate consistent: Child/carer experiences distress/upset/concern/frustration/ anger/embarrassment/withdrawal/severe depression/apathy in unfamiliar situations. Frequent emotional encouragement and support required.

3 Moderate frequent: Child/carer experiences distress/upset/concern/frustration/ anger/embarrassment/withdrawal/severe depression/apathy. Controls emotions with assistance, emotionally dependent on some occasions, vulnerable to change in routine, etc., spontaneously uses methods to assist emotional control.

4 Mild occasional: Child/carer experiences distress/upset/concern/frustration/anger/ embarrassment/withdrawal/severe depression/apathy. Able to control feelings in most situations, generally well adjusted/stable (most of the time/most situations), occasional emotional support/encouragement needed.

5 Not inappropriate (behaves appropriately in situation): Distress/upset/concern/ frustration/anger/embarrassment/withdrawal/severe depression/apathy. Well adjusted, stable and able to cope emotionally with most situations.

21 Dietetic Intervention for Undernutrition: Adults

Identify descriptor that is 'best fit'. The patient/client/student does not have to have each feature mentioned. Use 0.5 to indicate if patient/client/student is slightly better or worse than a descriptor and as appropriate to age.

Impairment

0 BMI <14kg/m^2 : Unintentional weight loss of more than 15% in past 3-6 months, significantly underweight and/or no oral intake for 5 days or more.

1 Unintentional weight loss of more than 10% in past 3-6 months and significantly underweight and/or currently meeting approximately 20% of nutritional needs.

2 Unintentional weight loss of more than 10% in past 3-6 months and/or currently meeting approximately 40% of nutritional needs.

3 Unintentional weight loss of more than 5% in past 3-6 months and/or currently meeting approximately 60% of nutritional needs.

4 Unintentional weight loss 0-5% in past 3-6 months and/or currently meeting approximately 80% of nutritional needs.

5 Healthy weight: BMI >18.5kg/m^2. No recent unintentional weight loss and meeting nutritional needs.

Activity

0 Full assistance needed for eating or drinking. Reliant on carers to prepare all meals, drinks and snacks. No appetite. No willingness to eat.

1 Needs a considerable amount of assistance to eat and drink. Can manage some finger foods, with supervision. Requires full assistance to prepare meals, drinks and snacks. Very reduced appetite. Mostly unwilling to eat.

2 May need some assistance when eating or drinking. Can manage all finger foods. Requires some assistance to prepare meals, drinks and snacks. Reduced appetite. Frequently unwilling to eat.

3 Able to prepare a meal, drink or snack with some assistance or adaptations. Able to eat or drink independently, with some support such as prompting or adaptations. Requires supervision to prepare meals, drinks and snacks. Variable appetite. Occasionally unwilling to eat.

4 Able to eat or drink independently with adaptations. Able to prepare meals, drinks and snacks with minimal supervision. Occasional suppressed appetite. Willing to eat.

5 Able to eat and drink independently. Able to prepare meals, drinks and snacks independently. Has a full appetite. Willing to eat.

Participation

0 No autonomy, isolated, no social family role.

1 Very limited choices, contact mainly with professionals, no social or family role, little control over life, limited ability to make lifestyle choices, food choices, treatment options.

2 Some integration, value and autonomy in one setting.

3 Integrated, valued and has autonomy in limited number of settings

4 Occasionally some restriction in autonomy, integration or role, can do things independently but has some barriers.

5 Integrated, valued, occupies appropriate role, takes responsibility for own health.

Wellbeing/Distress (client/carer)

0 Severe constant: High and constant levels of distress/upset/concern/frustration/anger/embarrassment/withdrawal/severe depression/apathy. Unable to express or control emotions appropriately.

1 Frequently severe: Moderate distress/upset/concern/frustration/anger/embarrassment/withdrawal/severe depression/apathy. Becomes concerned easily, requires constant reassurance/support, needs clear/tight limits and structure and loses emotional control easily.

2 Moderate consistent: Distress/upset/concern/frustration/anger/embarrassment/withdrawal/severe depression/apathy in unfamiliar situations, frequent emotional encouragement and support required.

3 Moderate frequent: Distress/upset/concern/frustration/anger/embarrassment/withdrawal/severe depression/apathy. Controls emotions with assistance, emotionally dependent on some occasions, vulnerable to change in routine, etc., spontaneously uses methods to assist emotional control.

4 Mild occasional: Distress/upset/concern/frustration/anger/embarrassment/withdrawal/ severe depression/apathy. Able to control feelings in most situations, generally well adjusted/stable (most of the time/most situations), occasional emotional support/ encouragement needed.

5 Not inappropriate (behaves appropriately in situation): Distress/upset/concern/ frustration/anger/embarrassment/withdrawal/severe depression/apathy. Well adjusted, stable and able to cope emotionally with most situations, good insight, accepts and understands own limitations.

22 Dysarthria

Identify descriptor that is 'best fit'. The patient/client/student does not have to have each feature mentioned. Use 0.5 to indicate if patient/client/student is slightly better or worse than a descriptor and as appropriate to age.

Impairment

0 Profound dysarthria. Severe persistent articulatory/prosodic impairment. Inability to produce any distinguishable speech sounds. No oral motor control. No respiratory support for speech.

1 Severe/moderate dysarthria. With consistent articulatory/prosodic impairment. Mostly open vowel sounds with some consonant approximations/severe festination of speech. Extremely effortful or slow speech; only 1 or 2 words per breath. Severely limited motor control.

2 Moderate dysarthria. With frequent episodes of articulatory/prosodic impairment. Most consonants attempted but poorly represented acoustically/moderate festination. Very slow speech; manages up to 4 words per breath. Moderate limitation oral motor control.

3 Moderate/mild dysarthria. Consistent omission/articulation of consonants. Variability of speed. Mild limitation of oral motor control or prosodic impairment.

4 Mild dysarthria. Slight or occasional omission/mispronunciation of consonants. Slight or occasional difficulty with oral motor control/prosody or respiratory support.

5 No impairment.

Activity

0 Unable to communicate in any way. No effective communication. No interaction.

1 Occasionally able to make basic needs known with familiar persons or trained listeners in familiar contexts. Minimal communication with maximal assistance.

2 Limited functional communication. Consistently able to make basic needs/conversation understood but is heavily dependent on cues and context. Communicates better with trained listener or family members or in familiar settings. Frequent repetition required. Maintained meaningful interaction related to here and now.

3 Consistently able to make needs known but can sometimes convey more information than this. Some inconsistency in unfamiliar settings. Is less dependent for intelligibility on cues and context. Occasional repetition required. Communicates beyond here/now with familiar persons, needs some cues and prompting.

4 Can be understood most of the time by any listener despite communication irregularities. Holds conversation, requires special consideration, for example, patience, time, attention, especially with a wider range of people.

5 Communicates effectively in all situations.

Participation

0 Unable to fulfil any social/educational/family role. Not involved in decision making/ no autonomy/no control over environment, no social integration.

1 Very limited choices, contact mainly with professionals, no social or family role, little control over life, limited ability to make lifestyle choices, food choices, treatment options.

2 Some self-confidence/some social integration. Makes some decisions and influences control in familiar situations.

3 Some self-confidence; autonomy emerging. Makes decisions and has control of some aspects of life. Able to achieve some limited social integration/educational activities. Diffident over control over life. Needs encouragement to achieve potential.

4 Mostly confident; occasional difficulties integrating or in fulfilling social/role activity. Participates in all appropriate decisions. May have difficulty in achieving potential in some situations occasionally.

5 Achieving potential. Autonomous and unrestricted. Able to fulfil social, educational and family role. Takes responsibility for own health.

Wellbeing/Distress (client/carer)

0 Severe constant: High and constant levels of distress/upset/concern/frustration/ anger/embarrassment/withdrawal/severe depression/apathy. Unable to express or control emotions appropriately.

1 Frequently severe: Moderate distress/upset/concern/frustration/anger/embarrassment/ withdrawal/severe depression/apathy. Becomes concerned easily, requires constant reassurance/support, needs clear/tight limits and structure, loses emotional control easily.

2 Moderate consistent: Distress/upset/concern/frustration/anger/embarrassment/ withdrawal/severe depression/apathy in unfamiliar situations. Frequent emotional encouragement and support required.

3 Moderate frequent: Distress/upset/concern/frustration/anger/embarrassment/ withdrawal/severe depression/apathy. Controls emotions with assistance, emotionally dependent on some occasions, vulnerable to change in routine, etc., spontaneously uses methods to assist emotional control.

4 Mild occasional: Distress/upset/concern/frustration/anger/embarrassment/withdrawal/ severe depression/apathy. Able to control feelings in most situations, generally well adjusted/stable (most of the time/most situations), occasional emotional support/ encouragement needed.

5 Not inappropriate: Distress/upset/concern/frustration/anger/embarrassment/ withdrawal/severe depression/apathy. Well adjusted, stable and able to cope emotionally with most situations, good insight, accepts and understands own limitations.

23 Dysfluency

Identify descriptor that is 'best fit'. The patient/client/student does not have to have each feature mentioned. Use 0.5 to indicate if patient/client/student is slightly better or worse than a descriptor and as appropriate to age.

Impairment

0 Profound stammer. Examples of behaviour: tension-associated gestures and behaviours, many repetitions, long prolongations, marked and repeated blocks; frequent avoidance of many words, stammer always evident.

1 Severe/moderate stammer. Examples of behaviour: blocks, fairly long prolongations, some tension-associated behaviours and gestures, occasional associated gestures and behaviours; frequent avoidance of some words, stammer frequently evident and severe stammer behaviours occurring occasionally.

2 Moderate stammering. Examples of behaviour: blocks, short prolongations, repetitions, some tension-associated behaviours and gestures; occasional avoidance of a few words, stammer sometimes evident or severe/moderate stammer occurring occasionally.

3 Moderate/slight stammer. Examples of behaviour: occasional prolongations, repetitions, slight tension; occasional avoidance of specific words, stammer sometimes evident or moderate stammer occurring occasionally.

4 Slight stammer. Examples of behaviour: easy repetitions; stammer occasionally evident or moderate stammer or avoidance occurring infrequently.

5 No stammer. Normal fluency.

Activity

0 Interaction severely disrupted at all times. Great difficulty getting message across to any listener.

1 Interaction severely disrupted with less familiar listeners in most situations, occasionally less disrupted with familiar listeners. Significant difficulty getting message across to listeners. Avoids many situations and people.

2 Interaction moderately disrupted with some listeners or in several different situations, less disrupted with other listeners/some difficulty getting message across to listener/ marked variability. Avoids some situations and people.

3 Interaction slightly disrupted with some listeners or situations, less disrupted with other listeners/slight difficulty getting message across to listener/less variability. Avoids occasional situations and people.

4 Interaction occasionally disrupted with some listeners or in occasional specific situations; no/very occasional problems with other listeners and slight difficulty getting message across to listener. Does not avoid situations or people.

5 No disruption to communication. No difficulty getting message across to listener.

Participation

0 Unable to fulfil any social/educational/family role. Not involved in decision making/ no autonomy/no control over environment, no social integration.

1 Low self-confidence/poor self-esteem/limited social integration/socially isolated/ contributes to some basic and limited decisions. Cannot achieve potential in any situation.

2 Some self-confidence/some social integration/makes some decisions and influences control in familiar situations.

3 Some self-confidence; autonomy emerging. Makes decisions and has control of some aspects of life. Able to achieve some limited social integration/educational activities. Diffident over control over life. Needs encouragement to achieve potential.

4 Mostly confident; occasional difficulties integrating or in fulfilling social/role activity. Participates in all appropriate decisions. May have difficulty in achieving potential in some situations occasionally.

5 Achieving potential. Autonomous and unrestricted. Able to fulfil social, educational and family role.

Wellbeing/Distress (client/carer)

0 Severe constant: High and constant levels of distress/upset/concern/frustration/ anger/embarrassment/withdrawal/severe depression/apathy. Unable to express or control emotions appropriately.

1 Frequently severe: Moderate distress/upset/concern/frustration/anger/embarrassment/ withdrawal/severe depression/apathy. Becomes concerned easily, requires constant reassurance/support, needs clear/tight limits and structure, loses emotional control easily.

2 Moderate consistent: Distress/upset/concern/frustration/anger/embarrassment/ withdrawal/severe depression/apathy in unfamiliar situations. Frequent emotional encouragement and support required.

3 Moderate frequent: Distress/upset/concern/frustration/anger/embarrassment/ withdrawal/severe depression/apathy. Controls emotions with assistance, emotionally dependent on some occasions, vulnerable to change in routine, etc., spontaneously uses methods to assist emotional control.

4 Mild occasional: Distress/upset/concern/frustration/anger/embarrassment/withdrawal/ severe depression/apathy. Able to control feelings in most situations, generally well adjusted/stable (most of the time/most situations), occasional emotional support/ encouragement needed.

5 Not inappropriate: Distress/upset/concern/frustration/anger/embarrassment/ withdrawal/severe depression/apathy. Well adjusted, stable and able to cope emotionally with most situations, good insight, accepts and understands own limitations.

24 Dysphagia

Identify descriptor that is 'best fit' The patient/client/student does not have to have each feature mentioned. Use 0.5 to indicate if patient/client/student is slightly better or worse than a descriptor and as appropriate to age.
Please note: minor changes to wording to the one recorded in 2015

Impairment

0 Profound. Aphagia: Not safe to swallow due to cognitive status/no bolus control/ aspiration/absence of oral/pharyngeal swallow. Aspiration risk identified on all consistencies with clinical signs of aspiration. No effective cough reflex. Not able to manage oral secretions. May need regular suction.

1 Severe dysphagia. Weak oral movements/no bolus control/inadequate/inconsistent swallow reflex. High and constant risk of aspiration on some but not all consistencies or daily. Can occasionally manage oral secretions

2 Severe/moderate dysphagia. Cough/swallow reflexes evident but abnormal or delayed. Uncoordinated oral movements. At regular risk of aspiration (several times a week). Difficulty managing oral secretions in some positions or at some times of the day.

3 Moderate dysphagia. Swallow and cough reflex present. May have poor oral control. At occasional risk of aspiration. Occasional difficulty with managing oral secretions.

4 Mild oral/pharyngeal dysphagia. Incoordination but no clinical risk or evidence of aspiration. No difficulty with managing oral secretions.

5 No evidence of dysphagia.

Activity

0 Unable to safely take any fluid/diet/modified consistencies. Unable to manage oral secretions. Needs experienced and constant surveillance. Requires non-oral methods to meet all hydration and nutritional needs. This may or may not be advised to be in the patient's interests by the responsible clinician and multidisciplinary team.

1 Oral intake insufficient to meet hydration and nutritional needs. Requires non-oral methods to meet all hydration and nutritional needs feeding or supplements. Occasionally able to take small amounts of food or drink/modified consistencies using compensatory strategies. Constantly refuses oral intake or holds bolus in the mouth. Requires experienced assistance, prompting and supervision. Requires non-oral methods to meet all hydration and nutritional needs. This may or may not be advised to be in the patient's interests by the responsible clinician and multidisciplinary team.

2 Additional non-oral nutrition, hydration or supplements needed. Consistently able to take small amounts of small amounts of food or drink/modified consistencies using compensatory strategies. Frequently refuses oral intake or holds bolus in the mouth. Needs experienced assistance, prompting and supervision.

3 Oral intake sufficient to meet hydration and nutrition needs but may require supplements. Consistently able to take modified consistencies using compensatory strategies. May occasionally refuse oral intake but responds to encouragement. Needs some supervision/encouragement. May eat extremely slowly.

4 Although eating and drinking is abnormal, it is good enough to meet nutritional requirements. No assistance/supervision required. No alternative or supplement feeding required. May take extra time and avoid certain foods, drinks, or eating situations.

5 Functionally eating and drinking a normal diet.

Participation

0 Unable to fulfil any social/ educational/ family role. Not involved in decision making/ no autonomy/no control over environment, no social integration.

1 Low self-confidence/poor self-esteem/limited social integration/socially isolated/ contributes to some basic and limited decisions. Cannot achieve potential in any situation.

2 Some self-confidence/some social integration/makes some decisions and influences control in familiar situations.

3 Some self-confidence; autonomy emerging. Makes decisions and has control of some aspects of life. Able to achieve some limited social integration/educational activities. Diffident over control over life. Needs encouragement to achieve potential.

4 Mostly confident; occasional difficulties integrating or in fulfilling social/role activity. Participates in all appropriate decisions. May have difficulty in achieving potential in some situations occasionally.

5 Achieving potential. Autonomous and unrestricted. Able to fulfil social, educational and family role.

Wellbeing/Distress (client/carer)

0 Severe constant: High and constant levels of distress/upset/concern/frustration/ anger/embarrassment/withdrawal/severe depression or apathy. Unable to express or control emotions appropriately.

1 Frequently severe: Moderate distress/upset/concern/frustration/anger/embarrassment/ withdrawal/severe depression or apathy. Becomes concerned easily, requires constant reassurance/support, needs clear/tight limits and structure, loses emotional control easily.

2 Moderate consistent: Distress/upset/concern/frustration/anger/embarrassment/ withdrawal/severe depression or apathy in unfamiliar situations. Frequent emotional encouragement and support required.

3 Moderate frequent: Distress/upset/concern/frustration/anger/embarrassment/ withdrawal/severe depression or apathy. Controls emotions with assistance, emotionally dependent on some occasions, vulnerable to change in routine, etc., spontaneously uses methods to assist emotional control.

4 Mild occasional: Distress/upset/concern/frustration/anger/embarrassment/withdrawal/ severe depression or apathy. Able to control feelings in most situations, generally well adjusted/stable (most of the time/most situations), occasional emotional support/ encouragement needed.

5 Not inappropriate: Distress/upset/concern/frustration/anger/embarrassment/ withdrawal/severe depression or apathy. Well adjusted, stable and able to cope emotionally with most situations, good insight, accepts and understands own limitations.

25 Dysphasia/Aphasia

Identify descriptor that is 'best fit'. The patient/client/student does not have to have each feature mentioned. Use 0.5 to indicate if patient/client/student is slightly better or worse than a descriptor and as appropriate to age.

Impairment

0 Profound. Aphasia affecting all modalities, auditory and reading comprehension inconsistent even at one keyword. No meaningful expression.

1 Severe dysphasia/aphasia: Auditory and/or reading comprehension is consistent at one keyword level. Occasionally understands and expresses limited amount within context.

2 Severe/moderate dysphasia/aphasia: Auditory and/or reading comprehension consistent at a minimum of two or three keyword level. Some limited verbal and/or written expression used appropriately and purposefully.

3 Moderate dysphasia/aphasia: Constant auditory and/or reading comprehension for simple sentences or structures. Inconsistent with complex commands and structures. Consistently reduced verbal and/or written language structure and vocabulary. May have a specific, more severe difficulty in one modality.

4 Mild dysphasia/aphasia: Occasional difficulties present in auditory and/or reading comprehension and in verbal and/or written expression particularly in more complex environments.

5 No dysphasia/aphasia.

Activity

0 Unable to communicate in any way. No effective communication. No interaction.

1 Occasionally able to make basic needs known with familiar persons or trained listeners in familiar contexts. Minimal communication with maximal assistance.

2 Limited functional communication. Consistently able to make basic needs/conversation understood but is heavily dependent on cues and context. Communicates better with trained listener or family members or in familiar settings. Frequent repetition required. Maintains meaningful interaction related to here and now.

3 Consistently able to make needs known but can sometimes convey more information than this. Some inconsistency in unfamiliar settings. Is less dependent for intelligibility on cues and context. Occasional repetition required. Communicates beyond here/now with familiar persons; needs cues and prompting.

4 Can be understood most of the time by any listener despite communication irregularities. Holds conversation; requires occasional prompts particularly with a wider range of people.

5 Communicates effectively in all situations.

Participation

0 Unable to fulfil any social/educational/family role. Not involved in decision making/ no autonomy/no control over environment; no social integration.

1 Low self-confidence/poor self-esteem/limited social integration/socially isolated/ contributes to some basic and limited decisions. Cannot achieve potential in any situation.

2 Some self-confidence/some social integration/makes some decisions and influences control in familiar situations.

3 Some self-confidence; autonomy emerging. Makes decisions and has control of some aspects of life. Able to achieve some limited social integration/educational activities. Diffident over control over life. Needs encouragement to achieve potential.

4 Mostly confident; occasional difficulties integrating or in fulfilling social/role activity. Participating in all appropriate decisions. May have difficulty in achieving potential in some situations occasionally.

5 Achieving potential. Autonomous and unrestricted. Able to fulfil social, educational and family role.

Wellbeing/Distress (client/carer)

0 Severe constant: High and constant levels of distress/upset/concern/frustration/ anger/embarrassment/withdrawal/severe depression/apathy. Unable to express or control emotions appropriately.

1 Frequently severe: Moderate distress/upset/concern/frustration/anger/embarrassment/ withdrawal/severe depression/apathy. Becomes concerned easily, requires constant reassurance/support, needs clear/tight limits and structure, loses emotional control easily.

2 Moderate consistent: Distress/upset/concern/frustration/anger/embarrassment/ withdrawal/severe depression/apathy in unfamiliar situations. Frequent emotional encouragement and support required.

3 Moderate frequent: Distress/upset/concern/frustration/anger/embarrassment/ withdrawal/severe depression/apathy. Controls emotions with assistance, emotionally dependent on some occasions, vulnerable to change in routine, etc., spontaneously uses methods to assist emotional control.

4 Mild occasional: Distress/upset/concern/frustration/anger/embarrassment/withdrawal/ severe depression/apathy. Able to control feelings in most situations, generally well adjusted/stable (most of the time/most situations), occasional emotional support/ encouragement needed.

5 Not inappropriate: Distress/upset/concern/frustration/anger/embarrassment/ withdrawal/severe depression/apathy. Well adjusted, stable and able to cope emotionally with most situations, good insight, accepts and understands own limitations.

26 Dysphonia

Identify descriptor that is 'best fit'. The patient/client/student does not have to have each feature mentioned. Use 0.5 to indicate if patient/client/student is slightly better or worse than a descriptor and as appropriate to age.

Impairment

0 Profound. Severe persistent aphonia. Unable or does not phonate.

1 Severe consistent dysphonia. Occasional phonation. May be dysphonic with aphonic episodes.

2 Moderate dysphonia. Can phonate but frequent episodes of marked vocal impairment.

3 Moderate/mild dysphonia. Less frequent episodes of dysphonia, for example occurs some time each day/or slight persistent 'huskiness'.

4 Mild dysphonia. Occasional episodes of dysphonia occurring, for example on a weekly basis or less.

5 No dysphonia. Appropriate/modal voice consistently used.

Activity

0 Voice production is completely ineffective/inappropriate in all situations.

1 Voice production is completely ineffective/inappropriate in most situations except occasionally with familiar listeners or modified environments.

2 Voice production is effective/appropriate in modified environments only, for example quiet or familiar situations.

3 Voice production is effective/appropriate but can be unpredictable in some situations. Voice production requires less personal attention and effort in most situations.

4 Voice production is effective/appropriate on most occasions. Rarely effortful. Very occasional difficulties experienced.

5 Voice production is spontaneously effective and appropriate.

Participation

0 Unable to fulfil any social/educational/family role. Not involved in decision making/ no autonomy/no control over environment/no social integration.

1 Low self-confidence/poor self-esteem/limited social integration/socially isolated/ contributes to some basic and limited decisions. Cannot achieve potential in any situation.

2 Some self-confidence/some social integration/makes some decisions and influences control in familiar situations.

3 Some self-confidence; autonomy emerging. Makes decisions and has control of some aspects of life. Able to achieve some limited social integration/educational activities. Diffident over control over life. Needs encouragement to achieve potential.

4 Mostly confident; occasional difficulties integrating or in fulfilling social/role activity. Participating in all appropriate decisions. May have difficulty in achieving potential in some situations occasionally.

5 Achieving potential. Autonomous and unrestricted. Able to fulfil social, educational and family role.

Wellbeing/Distress (client/carer)

0 Severe constant: High and constant levels of distress/upset/concern/frustration/ anger/embarrassment/withdrawal/severe depression/apathy, unable to express or control emotions appropriately.

1 Frequently severe: Moderate distress/upset/concern/frustration/anger/embarrassment/ withdrawal/severe depression/apathy. Becomes concerned easily, requires constant reassurance/support, needs clear/tight limits and structure, loses emotional control easily.

2 Moderate consistent: Distress/upset/concern/frustration/anger/embarrassment/ withdrawal/severe depression/apathy in unfamiliar situations, frequent emotional encouragement and support required.

3 Moderate frequent: Distress/upset/concern/frustration/anger/embarrassment/ withdrawal/severe depression/apathy. Controls emotions with assistance, emotionally dependent on some occasions, vulnerable to change in routine, etc., spontaneously uses methods to assist emotional control.

4 Mild occasional: Distress/upset/concern/frustration/anger/embarrassment/withdrawal/ severe depression/apathy. Able to control feelings in most situations, generally well adjusted/stable (most of the time/most situations), occasional emotional support/ encouragement needed.

5 Not inappropriate: Distress/upset/concern/frustration/anger/embarrassment/ withdrawal/severe depression/apathy. Well adjusted, stable and able to cope emotionally with most situations, good insight, accepts and understands own limitations.

27 Dyspraxia: Developmental Coordination Difficulties

Identify descriptor that is 'best fit'. The patient/client/student does not have to have each feature mentioned. Use 0.5 to indicate if patient/client/student is slightly better or worse than a descriptor and as appropriate to age.

Impairment

0 Profound problems evident in all areas of sensory-motor development including vestibular, sensory processing and modulation, movement and task planning and organization, balance and coordination. Severe perceptual and ideational difficulties. Severe generalized/motor impairment. Very limited attention to tasks.

1 Severe problems usually involving all areas as indicated above, or maybe involving severe problems in two or more areas or one profound overriding problem, for example severe sensory defensiveness or motor impairment.

2 Severe/moderate impairment in some areas, may involve one severe overriding area, for example gross or fine motor skills, perception, coordination, handwriting or movement planning.

3 Moderate impairment in some areas and/or specific moderate problems in one area, such as motor skills, organization, concentration, writing or perception.

4 Mild impairment in one or more areas involving fine or gross motor skills, perception, coordination, attention, praxis.

5 Age-appropriate motor and perceptual development in all areas.

Activity

0 Unable to function independently in any way. Unable to perform any activity without skilled and continual assistance, specialized equipment, supervision or simplification.

1 Occasionally able to perform some simple/automatic activities independently, or to perform some small parts of some tasks alone. Minimal function with maximum assistance.

2 Able to perform basic simple tasks or parts of more complex tasks. Works better with a familiar adult or family member, but lacks confidence or ability in unfamiliar situations. Difficulty learning new skills or transferring them to different situations. Verbal prompts help.

3 Consistently able to perform simple tasks or parts of more complex ones without help. Can occasionally attempt new tasks building on existing skills. Needs help for some activities, or extra time, or tasks to be broken down or simplified. Verbal prompting may be needed.

4 Occasional difficulties experienced in certain situations or with certain activities. May require extra time to complete tasks. Occasional verbal prompts may be helpful.

5 Functions well in all situations and is fully independent at an age-appropriate level.

Participation

0 Unable to fulfil any social/educational/family role. Not involved in decision making/ no autonomy/no control over environment, no social integration.

1 Low self-confidence/poor self-esteem/limited social integration/socially isolated/ contributes to some basic and limited decisions. Cannot achieve potential in any situation.

2 Some self-confidence/some social integration/makes some decisions and influences control in familiar situations.

3 Some self-confidence; autonomy emerging. Makes decisions and has control of some aspects of life. Able to achieve some limited social integration/educational activities. Diffident over control over life. Needs encouragement to achieve potential.

4 Mostly confident; occasional difficulties integrating or in fulfilling social/role activity. Participates in all appropriate decisions. May have difficulty in achieving potential in some situations occasionally.

5 Achieving potential. Autonomous and unrestricted. Able to fulfil social, educational and family role.

Wellbeing/Distress (client/carer)

0 Severe constant: High and constant levels of distress/upset/concern/frustration/ anger/embarrassment/withdrawal/severe depression/apathy. Unable to express or control emotions appropriately.

1 Frequently severe: Moderate distress/upset/concern/frustration/anger/embarrassment/ withdrawal/severe depression/apathy. Becomes concerned easily, requires constant reassurance/support, needs clear/tight limits and structure, loses emotional control easily.

2 Moderate consistent: Distress/upset/concern/frustration/anger/embarrassment/ withdrawal/severe depression/apathy in unfamiliar situations, frequent emotional encouragement and support required.

3 Moderate frequent: Distress/upset/concern/frustration/anger/embarrassment/ withdrawal/severe depression/apathy. Controls emotions with assistance, emotionally dependent on some occasions, vulnerable to change in routine, etc., spontaneously uses methods to assist emotional control.

4 Mild occasional: Distress/upset/concern/frustration/anger/embarrassment/withdrawal/ severe depression/apathy. Able to control feelings in most situations, generally well adjusted/stable (most of the time/most situations), occasional emotional support/ encouragement needed.

5 Not inappropriate: Distress/upset/concern/frustration/anger/embarrassment/ withdrawal/severe depression/apathy. Well adjusted, stable and able to cope emotionally with most situations, good insight, accepts and understands own limitations.

28 Equipment Services

Identify the descriptor that is 'best fit'. The person rated does not need to have each feature mentioned. Use 0.5 to indicate if patient/client is likely to be better or worse than the descriptor. You may choose to give a carer a 'wellbeing' score if that is appropriate to your care plan.

Complete each of the impairment scores: physical, cognitive, sensory, speech, language (using the scales to guide you).

If the equipment is to improve physical independence, use this adapted scale. If the equipment provided is to address communication difficulties, use the AAC adapted scale.

Impairment (5 scores)	Activity (2 scores)		Participation (1 score)	Wellbeing (1 score)	Carer wellbeing (1 score if relevant)
Physical	Without equipment				
Cognitive	With equipment				
Sensory					
Speech and Language Output					
Comp-rehension					

Impairment: Physical

0 Profound abnormality of tone/control/movement, with total body involvement. No voluntary control over any movement.

1 Severe abnormality of tone/control/movement, with total body involvement. Minimal voluntary control of movement.

2 Moderate abnormality of tone/control/movement, with total body involvement or the severe involvement of two limbs. Some reliable movement or gross voluntary control of movement which may be uncoordinated, very slow or disrupted

3 Moderate abnormality of tone/control/movement, with partial involvement or severe single limb involvement. Impaired voluntary control of movement, which may be inaccurate and slow.

4 Mild abnormality of tone/control/movement, with mild impairment in voluntary control of movement and control. May have occasional incoordination and inaccuracies.

5 No physical impairment.

Impairment: Cognitive

0 Unresponsive to stimuli.

1 Non-purposeful random and fragmented responses. Occasional response to some simple commands; responses may be severely delayed or inappropriate. RecogniZes familiar people and routine tasks in context. Cooperates occasionally. Shows little sign of recall/memory. Can learn simple routines/tasks with maximal assistance.

2 Inconsistent reactions directly related to type of stimulus presented. Occasionally responds appropriately. Response may be delayed but appropriate. Recognizes familiar people in more settings. Can attend but is highly distractible. Unable to focus on individual tasks. Memory may be severely impaired; may perform a few simple learned tasks within familiar structure/setting. Insight, judgement and problem-solving are poor.

3 Recognizes familiar people and tasks in most contexts, able to retain small amounts of information consistently. Responds appropriately with some consistency. Appears orientated to setting. Insight, judgement and problem-solving are sometimes unreliable.

4 Alert and able to learn but needs occasional prompting and assistance. Responds well in most situations. Able to recall and integrate past and recent events. Shows carryover for new learning and when activities are learned. Good insight and judgement. May have problems with abstract reasoning in unusual circumstances. Occasional minor memory problem.

5 No cognitive impairment. Good insight, judgement and problem-solving abilities. Responds appropriately. Is alert and able to learn.

Impairment: Sensory

(Rate the person wearing glasses and hearing aids if normally used)

0 Profound hearing and visual impairment.

1 Severe hearing or visual impairment. Can perceive very restricted range of environmental sights or sounds. Limited benefit from hearing aid/glasses.

2 Severe/moderate hearing or visual impairment. Requires attention to perceive a limited range of sights and/or sounds. Benefits from hearing aid/glasses.

3 Moderate hearing or visual impairment. Can hear/see a range of environmental sounds and sights. Benefits greatly from hearing aid/glasses.

4 Mild hearing or visual impairment. Occasional difficulty with hearing in some environments or seeing in some lights. Benefits greatly from hearing aid/glasses

5 No hearing or visual impairment.

Impairment: Speech and language

Output without AAC; you may be helped by reviewing the impairment scales associated with SLI, dysarthria, dysphasia, ASD, etc.

0 Profound presentation of this impairment.

1 Severe presentation of this impairment.

2 Severe/moderate presentation of this impairment.

3 Moderate presentation of this impairment.

4 Mild presentation of this impairment.

5 No impairment.

Impairment: Comprehension

0 Profound difficulty. Comprehension inconsistent even at one keyword level in context.

1 Severe difficulty. Understanding limited to few recogniZable words in context or accompanied by visual clues, context, etc.

2 Severe/moderate comprehension difficulty. Can comprehend in familiar context, but inconsistent in ability. Familiar topics of conversation, e.g., familiar names, greetings, basic instructions in context can usually be understood.

3 Moderate comprehension difficulty. Can understand simple sentences and structures, but has difficulty with quick changes of subject, more complex topics or understanding in some contexts when there may be distraction/noise.

4 Mild/occasional difficulty in comprehension. Generally understands most conversation but has difficulty understanding occasionally, e.g., when tired/stressed.

5 No difficulty in comprehending. Normal receptive ability.

Activity

0 Cannot perform any purposeful activity independently; totally dependent on others in all environments.

1 Able to perform limited activities (around 20% of desired activities with assistance, e.g., prompting, encouragement or physical). This includes activity with others, such as adjusting or controlling environment.

2 Able to perform some activities (around 40% of desired activities). Can undertake a few tasks independently, i.e., without assistance.

3 Able to perform a range of activities on own (around 60% of desired activities). Able to perform a range of activities independently, though help (e.g., prompting, encouragement or physical) is needed for some activities.

4 Able to perform most activities on own (around 80% of desired activities). Needs extra time/encouragement or uses strategies to perform at this level.

5 Able to perform all activities independently.

Participation

(Autonomy/self-sufficiency/self-reliance = able to determine and have control over one's own viewpoint and not have decisions made by others)

0 Unable to fulfil any social/occupational/family role. No autonomy. No control in the environment. No social integration.

1 Low self-confidence, poor self-esteem, limited social integration, socially isolated. Unable to fulfil any educational/occupational role. No friends/acquaintances outside family/carers. Only able to engage in social activities with large amounts of support from carers.

2 Some degree of self-confidence and social integration beyond immediate family and carers. Fulfilling some social occupational education or family role with support. Able to effect some decisions/control in familiar situations. Social life will be very limited.

3 Makes decisions and has control over some aspects of life. Able to engage with family/occupation/recreation/education system to some extent with appropriate adjustment and support. Has a few friends/acquaintances. Has some autonomy and control over life. Needs encouragement to achieve potential.

4 Autonomous in most or all activities. May have occasional difficulties integrating or in fulfilling social/role activity. May have difficulty in achieving potential in some situations on some occasions. May have restricted interests/pastimes.

5 Autonomous in all activities. Able to fulfil social, occupational and family role.

Wellbeing/Distress

(For example, are they more or less upset/distressed/frustrated without access to their EC equipment, or does this make little difference and they have the same emotional state with or without?)

0 High and constant levels of distress and problematic emotions, like frustration/elation/anger, etc. May have severe depression and/or severe anxiety. May have severe apathy/social withdrawal. Likely to be unable to express or control emotions appropriately.

1 Severe levels of distress and problematic emotions. These are present all or nearly all of the time. Becomes distressed easily, requires constant reassurance/support, needs clear/tight limits and structure, loses emotional control easily.

2 Moderate to severe levels of distress and problematic emotions. Present most of the time. Frequent emotional support required.

3 Moderate levels of distress and problematic emotions. Occur frequently, more likely to occur in novel situations/changes in routine. Controls emotions with assistance, emotionally dependent on some occasions, but can use strategies to assist emotional control.

4 Mild levels of distress and problematic emotions. Not present all the time, likely only associated with novel situations or changes of routine. Able to control feelings in most situations, generally well adjusted/stable (most of the time/most situations), and occasional emotional support needed.

5 Well adjusted, stable and able to cope emotionally with most situations. Good insight, accepts and understands own limitations.

Carer Wellbeing/Distress

Use if relevant. Some carers may find it is more upsetting/frustrating/anxiety producing when the individual is using technology whilst others may find the opposite.

0 High and constant levels of distress and problematic emotions, like frustration/elation/anger, etc. May have severe depression and/or severe anxiety. May have severe apathy/social withdrawal. Likely to be unable to express or control emotions appropriately.

1 Severe levels of distress and problematic emotions. These are present all or nearly all of the time. Becomes distressed easily, requires constant reassurance/support, needs clear/tight limits and structure, loses emotional control easily.

2 Moderate to severe levels of distress and problematic emotions. Present most of the time. Frequent emotional support required.

3 Moderate levels of distress and problematic emotions. Occur frequently, more likely to occur in novel situations/changes in routine. Controls emotions with assistance, emotionally dependent on some occasions, but can use strategies to assist emotional control.

4 Mild levels of distress and problematic emotions. Not present all the time, likely only associated with novel situations or changes of routine. Able to control feelings in most situations, generally well-adjusted/stable (most of the time/most situations), and occasional emotional support needed.

5 Well adjusted, stable and able to cope emotionally with most situations. Good insight, accepts and understands own limitations.

Acknowledgement: Graeme Marsh in collaboration with Environmental Controls Clinical Reference Group Environmental - Subgroup Working Party.

29 Head Injury

Identify descriptor that is 'best fit'. The patient/client/student does not have to have each feature mentioned. Use 0.5 to indicate if patient/client/student is slightly better or worse than a descriptor and as appropriate to age.

Impairment

0 Profound. Inability to respond to external stimuli/gross loss of passive range of movement affecting multiple joints. Debilitated, minimal muscle power, multi-joint contractures/swelling. Total flaccidity/severe spasticity. Severe continual involuntary movements. Total loss of righting and equilibrium reactions. Severe global symptoms.

1 Responsive but uncooperative, range of movement maximally restricted. Passive range of movement moderately restricted. Pain on passive movement. No standing balance. Unable to weight bear. Minimal controlled voluntary movement. Severe sensory inattention. Low tone/moderate spasticity. Strong associated reactions. Severe degree of several signs and symptoms, for example dense hemiplegia, poor trunk control and some perceptual deficit.

2 Range of movement moderately restricted. Pain on active movement. Poor static balance. Some controlled purposeful movement. Moderate to severe inattention. Moderate involuntary movement. Associated reactions occurring on preparation to movement.

3 Some active participation, active range of movement with minimal restriction. Some associated reactions during movement. Purposeful but not necessarily accurate voluntary movement. Moderate sensory inattention. Minimal involuntary movement. Intermittent pain on active movement. Poor dynamic standing balance. May have one severe sign or symptom alone, for example dense hemiplegia or severe perceptual deficit, or a combination of milder signs or symptoms, for example mild hemiparesis with some sensory loss and occasional incontinence.

4 Slight/minimal abnormality of strength, muscle tone, range of movement. Difficulty with balance, purposeful accurate voluntary movements. May have abnormal speed of movement, slight incoordination. Minimal associated reaction with efforts.

5 Age-appropriate strength, range of movement and coordination. Normal tone and active movements.

Activity

0 No purposeful active movement, totally dependent, requires full physical care and constant vigilant supervision. May have totally disruptive and uncooperative behaviour. Dependent on skilled assistance.

1 Bed/chair-bound but unable to sit independently. Some very limited purposeful activity. Needs high level of assistance in most tasks. Some awareness, some effort and recognition to contribute to care. Dependent on skilled assistance.

2 Head and trunk control. Limited self-help skills. Initiates some aspects of ADL. Transfers with one, mobilizes with two. Requires physical and verbal prompting and supervision for most tasks and movements. Participates in care and engages in some structured activity. Dependent on familiar assistant.

3 Transfers or walking requires supervision or help of one. Undertakes personal care in modified supported environment. Appropriately initiates activities and needs assistance or supervision with some unfamiliar or complex tasks. Initiates activities appropriately.

4 Carries out personal care and tasks but is less efficient (clumsy), requires extra time or may need encouragement, assistance with unfamiliar tasks. Minimal or occasional assistance required for some complex tasks.

5 Age-appropriate independence.

Participation

0 Unable to fulfil any social/educational/family role. Not involved in decision making/ no autonomy/no control over environment, no social integration.

1 Low self-confidence/poor self-esteem/limited social integration/socially isolated/ contributes to some basic and limited decisions. Cannot achieve potential in any situation.

2 Some self-confidence/some social integration/makes some decisions and influences control in familiar situations.

3 Some self-confidence; autonomy emerging. Makes decisions and has control of some aspects of life. Able to achieve some limited social integration/educational activities. Diffident over control over life. Needs encouragement to achieve potential.

4 Mostly confident; occasional difficulties integrating or in fulfilling social/role activity. Participates in all appropriate decisions. May have difficulty in achieving potential in some situations occasionally.

5 Achieving potential. Autonomous and unrestricted. Able to fulfil social, educational and family role.

Wellbeing/Distress (client/carer)

0 Severe constant: High and constant levels of distress/upset/concern/frustration/anger/embarrassment/withdrawal/severe depression/apathy. Unable to express or control emotions appropriately.

1 Frequently severe: Moderate distress/upset/concern/frustration/anger/embarrassment/withdrawal/severe depression/apathy. Becomes concerned easily, requires constant reassurance/support, needs clear/tight limits and structure, loses emotional control easily.

2 Moderate consistent: Distress/upset/concern/frustration/anger/embarrassment/withdrawal/severe depression/apathy in unfamiliar situations. Frequent emotional encouragement and support required.

3 Moderate frequent: Distress/upset/concern/frustration/anger/embarrassment/withdrawal/severe depression/apathy. Controls emotions with assistance, emotionally dependent on some occasions, vulnerable to change in routine, etc., spontaneously uses methods to assist emotional control.

4 Mild occasional: Distress/upset/concern/ frustration/anger/embarrassment/withdrawal/severe depression/apathy. Able to control feelings in most situations, generally well adjusted/stable (most of the time/most situations), occasional emotional support/encouragement needed.

5 Not inappropriate: Distress/upset/concern/frustration/anger/embarrassment/withdrawal/severe depression/apathy. Well adjusted, stable and able to cope emotionally with most situations, good insight, accepts and understands own limitations.

30 Hearing Impairment/Deafness*

You may wish to rate impairment twice: first without hearing aid and second with amplification (functional listening skills). You may wish to omit the independence with amplification if the patient/client/student is not aided or has made an informed decision to not use amplification.

Identify descriptor that is 'best fit'. The patient/client/student does not have to have each feature mentioned. Use 0.5 to indicate if patient/client/student is slightly better or worse than a descriptor and as appropriate to age. You may wish to rate impairment twice: first without hearing aid and second with hearing aid.

Impairment

0 Profound difficulties. Unable to detect or discriminate any speech or environmental sounds. Hears at 95 decibels or more.

1 Severe difficulties. Can perceive very restricted range of environmental and speech sounds. Hears at 70 to 94 decibels.

2 Severe/moderate difficulties. Requires attention to perceive a limited range of speech and environmental sounds. Hears at 40 to 69 decibels.

3 Moderate difficulties. Detects and discriminates a range of speech and environmental sounds. Hears at 25 to 39 decibels.

4 Mild difficulties. Unable to hear some specific frequencies; detects and discriminates most speech and environmental sounds.

5 No difficulties. Able to hear a full range of frequencies; detects and discriminates all speech and environmental sounds. Normal hearing.

Activity

0 No functional communication. Unable to communicate needs or preferences. Needs familiar or highly-trained people to identify possible indications of needs or preferences. Unable to hear very loud voice.

1 Limited functional communication with familiar people who are trained in meeting their communication needs. Adapted environments or communication modes required. Minimal communication with high levels of assistance.

2 Limited functional communication in familiar situations but needs a high level of support. Developing functional communication with familiar people. Able to make needs and preferences known approximately 50% of the time with medium levels of assistance. Communication breakdowns are frequent and difficulties with communication repair.

3 Functional communication in familiar situations but may need some verbal/physical assistance at other times. Consistent level of general functional communication with trained or familiar people. Able to make requests, comments and ask questions. Communication breakdowns continue to occur, especially if context is less familiar. Reliance on communication partner to facilitate communication repair.

4 Requires some minor assistance or extra time to communicate with others. Able to communicate effectively in most situations. May continue to present with mild difficulties when communicating complex ideas or with unfamiliar people. Attempts to repair communication breakdown.

5 Age appropriate – communicates well in all situations. Consistent effective communication in usual range of environments.

Participation

0 Unable to fulfil any social/educational/family role. No control over their environment or events/activities they are part of. Not involved in any decision making. Not integrated into their social settings or activities.

1 Low self-confidence/poor self-esteem/socially isolated. Some control over their environment or activities they are part of. Able to make some basic decisions. Unable to achieve potential in identified situations.

2 Some self-confidence/some social integration. Able to control and make decisions in familiar activities, environments or with familiar people. Can integrate into social settings or activities with a high level of support.

3 Some self-confidence; autonomy emerging. Confidence and decision making becoming more secure. Limited social integration or participation achieved with support. Needs encouragement to achieve potential in more challenging situations.

4 Mostly confident and can make decisions in most situations. Occasional difficulties integrating into a social setting or activity, and needs minimal support to overcome this. May experience some difficulties achieving potential in challenging situations.

5 Achieving potential in all areas. Able to participate in all social settings and activities. Is able to make decisions and exert control over all aspects of their life.

Wellbeing

0 Severe constant: High and constant levels of distress/upset/concern/frustration/anger/embarrassment/withdrawal/severe depression or apathy. Unable to express or control emotions appropriately in all situations. Very poor perception of self and sense of identity.

1 Frequently severe: Moderate levels of distress/upset/concern/frustration/anger/embarrassment/withdrawal/severe depression or apathy. Becomes concerned or agitated easily. Requires constant reassurance or support. Needs clear boundaries and structure. Loses emotional control easily. Poor perception of self and sense of identity.

2 Moderate consistent: Distress/upset/concern/frustration/anger/embarrassment/withdrawal/severe depression or apathy in unfamiliar situations. Frequent emotional encouragement and support required. Low self-image and identity; needs a high level of support.

3 Moderate frequent: Controls emotions on some occasions with support. Vulnerable to change in routine. Able to use methods to assist emotional control. Developing a positive self-image and identity; needs support.

4 Mild occasional: Able to control feelings in most situations. Generally emotionally stable or well adjusted. Occasionally requires emotional support/encouragement. Generally has a positive self-image and identity; needs occasional support.

5 Not inappropriate: Well adjusted, stable and able to cope emotionally with most situations. Good insight into their own emotions. Accepts and understands their limitations/needs. Positive self-image and identity.

Optional area

Independence with amplification

0 No use of amplification. Complete resistance to wearing aid/cochlear implant. Becomes highly distressed if aids or implants are attempted to be put on.

1 Limited use of amplification. Resists wearing aid/cochlear implant. Frequently avoids aids or implants being put on as well as pulling them off. Needs high level of distraction to wear aids/implants for short periods of time.

2 Wears aids/implants for longer periods of time. Needs distraction initially to put device on but then wears them for prolonged time without support. Unable to indicate fault with device.

3 Wears aids/implants consistently in some environments. Does not wear devices in all communication settings, e.g., home. Not consistently or delayed in indicating fault with device.

4 Consistent user of hearing aids/implants in relevant settings. Will request device. Needs support to indicate a fault with device.

5 Consistent user of hearing aids/implants in relevant settings. Can indicate if there are faults with device. Able to maintain aids independently or able to indicate if further support is required.

Acknowledgement: Helen Merry, Emily Beadle, Lisa Nash and the Acute Paediatric Speech and Language Therapy Team at the Royal London Children's Hospital.

31 Incontinence

Identify descriptor that is 'best fit'. The patient/client/student does not have to have each feature mentioned. Use 0.5 to indicate if patient/client/student is slightly better or worse than a descriptor and as appropriate to age.

Impairment

0 Profound. No muscle power; bladder/bowel instability; no sensation, severe bladder/bowel prolapse; severe continual pain.

1 Flicker of muscle contraction. Intermittent severe pain.

2 Weak muscle contraction/diminished sensation. Some moderate pain.

3 Muscle contraction but not maintained against gravity. Evidence of instability. Occasional pain.

4 Muscle contraction against gravity. No pain; minor degree of prolapse.

5 Full muscle power and tone/stable bladder and bowel; full sensation, no prolapse.

Activity

0 Total lack of voluntary control; inability to recognize the need for bowel/bladder evacuation. Constant use of pads.

1 Recognizes need to evacuate but inability to control.

2 Some ability to control bowel/bladder/frequency/urgency. Only manages with structured routine, able to go out for short periods with pads/toilet availability.

3 Intermittent bowel problems/frequent stress incontinence/urgency.

4 Very occasional stress incontinence (on laughing or coughing).

5 Normal bladder and bowel control.

Participation

0 Unable to fulfil any social/educational/family role. Not involved in decision making/no autonomy/no control over environment, no social integration.

1 Low self-confidence/poor self-esteem/limited social integration/socially isolated/ contributes to some basic and limited decisions. Cannot achieve potential in any situation.

2 Some self-confidence/some social integration/makes some decisions and influences control in familiar situations.

3 Some self-confidence; autonomy emerging. Makes decisions and has control of some aspects of life. Able to achieve some limited social integration/educational activities. Diffident over control over life. Needs encouragement to achieve potential.

4 Mostly confident; occasional difficulties integrating or in fulfilling social/role activity. Participates in all appropriate decisions. May have difficulty in achieving potential in some situations occasionally.

5 Achieving potential. Autonomous and unrestricted. Able to fulfil social, educational and family role.

Wellbeing/Distress (client/carer)

0 Severe constant: Upset/frustration/anger/distress/embarrassment/concern/withdrawal. High and constant levels of concern/anger/severe depression/apathy. Unable to express or control emotions appropriately.

1 Frequently severe: Upset/frustration/anger/distress/embarrassment/concern/ withdrawal. Moderate concern, becomes concerned easily, requires constant reassurance/ support, needs clear/tight limits and structure, loses emotional control easily.

2 Moderate consistent: Upset/frustration/anger/distress/embarrassment/concern/ withdrawal. Concern in unfamiliar situation, frequent emotional encouragement and support required.

3 Moderate frequent: Upset/frustration/anger/distress/embarrassment/concern/ withdrawal. Controls emotions with assistance, emotionally dependent on some occasions, vulnerable to change in routine, etc., spontaneously uses methods to assist emotional control.

4 Mild occasional: Upset/frustration/anger/distress/embarrassment/concern/withdrawal. Able to control feelings in most situations, generally well adjusted/stable (most of the time/most situations), occasional emotional support/encouragement needed.

5 Not inappropriate: Upset/frustration/anger/distress/embarrassment/concern/ withdrawal.

32 Laryngectomy

Identify descriptor that is 'best fit'. The patient/client/student does not have to have each feature mentioned. Use 0.5 to indicate if patient/client/student is slightly better or worse than a descriptor and as appropriate to age.

Impairment

0 Profound. Laryngectomy complicated by stomach pull or requiring skin grafting or colon transplant.

1 Laryngectomy complicated by poor healing, fistulae.

2 Uncomplicated laryngectomy, well healed.

3 Hemi-laryngectomy, removal of one cord and part of thyroid cartilage.

4 Removal of vocal cord or associated soft tissue only.

5 Normal larynx.

Activity

0 Pseudo voice production is completely ineffective in all situations.

1 Pseudo voice production is completely ineffective in most situations other than with a trained listener or in a modified environment.

2 Pseudo voice production is effective with attention of listener in modified environments, for example quiet situations, familiar situations. Requires considerable effort.

3 Pseudo voice is effective on certain occasions. Pseudo voice requires some personal effort all the time.

4 Pseudo voice is effective on most occasions. Slightly effortful. Able to use the telephone.

5 Pseudo voice is effective in all situations.

Participation

0 Unable to fulfil any social/educational/family role. Not involved in decision making/ no autonomy/no control over environment, no social integration.

1 Low self-confidence/poor self-esteem/limited social integration/socially isolated/ contributes to some basic and limited decisions. Cannot achieve potential in any situation.

2 Some self-confidence/some social integration/makes some decisions and influences control in familiar situations.

3 Some self-confidence; autonomy emerging. Makes decisions and has control of some aspects of life. Able to achieve some limited social integration/educational activities. Diffident over control over life. Needs encouragement to achieve potential.

4 Mostly confident; occasional difficulties integrating or in fulfilling social/role activity. Participates in all appropriate decisions. May have difficulty in achieving potential in some situations occasionally.

5 Achieving potential. Autonomous and unrestricted. Able to fulfil social, educational and family role.

Wellbeing/Distress (client/carer)

0 Severe constant: High and constant levels of distress/upset/concern/frustration/ anger/embarrassment/withdrawal/severe depression/apathy. Unable to express or control emotions appropriately.

1 Frequently severe: Moderate distress/upset/concern/frustration/anger/embarrassment/ withdrawal/severe depression/apathy. Becomes concerned easily, requires constant reassurance/support, needs clear/tight limits and structure, loses emotional control easily.

2 Moderate consistent: Distress/upset/concern/frustration/anger/embarrassment/ withdrawal/severe depression/apathy in unfamiliar situations, frequent emotional encouragement and support required.

3 Moderate frequent: Distress/upset/concern/frustration/anger/embarrassment/ withdrawal/severe depression/apathy. Controls emotions with assistance, emotionally dependent on some occasions, vulnerable to change in routine, etc., spontaneously uses methods to assist emotional control.

4 Mild occasional: Distress/upset/concern/frustration/anger/embarrassment/withdrawal/ severe depression/apathy. Able to control feelings in most situations, generally well adjusted/stable (most of the time/most situations), occasional emotional support/ encouragement needed.

5 Not inappropriate: Distress/upset/concern/frustration/anger/embarrassment/withdrawal/ severe depression/apathy. Well adjusted, stable and able to cope emotionally with most situations, good insight, accepts and understands own limitations.

33 Learning Disability: Communication

Identify descriptor that is 'best fit'. The patient/client/client does not have to have each feature mentioned. Use 0.5 to indicate if patient/client/student is slightly better or worse than a descriptor and as appropriate to age.

Impairment

0 Profound. Severe communication impairment. Multiple areas of impairment including speech/language, sensory and cognition. No communicative intent.

1 Severe/moderate communication impairment. Several areas of impairment: speech/language, sensory, cognition. May have some slight ability in one area, for example basic recognition.

2 Moderate communication impairment. Several areas of moderate impairment: speech/language, sensory, cognitive. There may be one severe overriding difficulty, for example severe articulatory disorder.

3 Moderate/slight communication impairment. One moderate impairment with speech/language/sensory or cognitive. Two or less areas of impairment.

4 Slight communication impairment. Slight impairment of speech/language, sensory or cognition.

5 No communication impairment.

Activity

0 Unable to communicate in any way. No effective understanding even in context.

1 Shows intentional communication but this is inconsistent. Occasionally able to make simple basic needs known and able to follow stage one instructions in context; can only do this with a trained communication partner in familiar settings. Minimal communication with maximal assistance.

2 Consistant but limited intentional communication. Limited functional communication. Consistently able to make basic needs known and able to follow simple instructions out of context. Communicates better with a trained listener and family members but can occasionally communicate basic needs with unknown people in familiar settings. Depends heavily on context and cues.

3 Consistently able to make basic needs known but can occasionally convey more information than this. Able to follow most everyday simple conversations in context; can communicate just as well with familiar people or strangers in some unfamiliar as well as familiar settings. Needs fewer cues and assistance.

4 Consistently able to convey information but has some difficulty conveying more abstract and complex thoughts. Able to understand almost all everyday conversation but still has occasional difficulty with complex information. Less context dependent.

5 Communicates well in all situations.

Participation

0 Unable to fulfil any social/educational/family role. Not involved in decision making/ no autonomy/no control over environment, no social integration.

1 Low self-confidence/poor self-esteem/limited social integration/socially isolated/ contributes to some basic and limited decisions. Cannot achieve potential in any situation.

2 Some self-confidence/some social integration/makes some decisions and influences control in familiar situations.

3 Some self-confidence; autonomy emerging. Makes decisions and has control of some aspects of life. Able to achieve some limited social integration/educational activities. Diffident over control over life. Needs encouragement to achieve potential.

4 Mostly confident; occasional difficulties integrating or in fulfilling social/role activity. Participates in all appropriate decisions. May have difficulty in achieving potential in some situations occasionally.

5 Achieving potential. Autonomous and unrestricted. Able to fulfil social, educational and family role.

Wellbeing/Distress (client/carer)

0 Severe constant: High and constant levels of distress/upset/concern/frustration/ anger/embarrassment/withdrawal/severe depression/apathy. Unable to express or control emotions appropriately.

1 Frequently severe: Moderate distress/upset/concern/frustration/anger/embarrassment/ withdrawal/severe depression/apathy. Becomes concerned easily, requires constant reassurance/support, needs clear/tight limits and structure, loses emotional control easily.

2 Moderate consistent: Distress/upset/concern/frustration/anger/embarrassment/ withdrawal/severe depression/apathy in unfamiliar situations. Frequent emotional encouragement and support required.

3 Moderate frequent: Distress/upset/concern/frustration/anger/embarrassment/ withdrawal/severe depression or apathy. Controls emotions with assistance, emotionally dependent on some occasions, vulnerable to change in routine, etc., spontaneously uses methods to assist emotional control.

4 Mild occasional: Distress/upset/concern/frustration/anger/embarrassment/withdrawal/ severe depression/apathy. Able to control feelings in most situations, generally well adjusted/stable (most of the time/most situations), occasional emotional support/ encouragement needed.

5 Not inappropriate: Distress/upset/concern/frustration/anger/embarrassment/ withdrawal/severe depression/apathy. Well adjusted, stable and able to cope emotionally with most situations, good insight, accepts and understands own limitations.

34 Mental Health

Identify descriptor that is 'best fit'. The patient/client/student does not have to have each feature mentioned. Use 0.5 to indicate if patient/client/student is slightly better or worse than a descriptor and as appropriate to age.

Impairment

0 Profound. Catatonic, unresponsive; no volition, persistent/severe and wide range of thought disorders, fixed delusions, persistent visual, auditory, tactile hallucinations, persistent/severe disturbance of affect. Severe memory loss. No insight.

1 Severe thought disorder, auditory hallucinations frequent, variable disturbances of affect, little volition. Occasionally past memories recalled. Some automatic response. Apathetic, no motivation, no initiation. Recognizes own name and that of some individuals and situations. No insight into confusion.

2 Moderate thought disorder in duration, severity, frequency, some auditory hallucinations present, moderate disturbance of affect, moderate level of volition, some remote memory. Inappropriate responses to some stimuli. Occasional partial insight.

3 Evidence of some thought disorder, occasional evidence of auditory/visual hallucination, usually stable mood, volition intact. Some recent memory. Some insight. Attempts to express feeling and 'sort things out'. Orientated in regular surroundings, easily confused.

4 Very occasional evidence of some thought disorder in duration, severity, frequency, good level insight, usually stable mood, volition intact. Occasionally disturbed by new or occasional complex experiences. Short-term memory deficit. Can express feeling. Very occasional disorientation.

5 Well developed insight, high-level volition, no evidence of thought disorder, delusion, hallucination. Appropriate memory. Orientated.

Activity

0 Inability to recognize body functions and requirement. May have totally disruptive and uncooperative behaviour. Totally dependent, requires full physical care and constant vigilant supervision.

1 Recognizes some bodily requirements and occasionally initiates actively but requires high level of assistance and supervision in most tasks.

2 Able to cooperate in self-care and relate to others in protected environment but is dependent on verbal prompting to initiate and continue tasks. Requires some physical assistance.

3 Needs occasional verbal prompting to initiate movement/care. Able to operate without supervision for short periods, able to have some independence with encouragement. Independent in familiar surroundings only.

4 Able to live independently with some occasional support, requires extra time, encouragement. Assistance occasionally required with unfamiliar tasks.

5 Age-appropriate independence.

Participation

0 Unable to fulfil any social/educational/family role. Not involved in decision making/no autonomy/no control over environment, no social integration.

1 Low self-confidence/poor self-esteem/limited social integration/socially isolated/contributes to some basic and limited decisions. Cannot achieve potential in any situation.

2 Some self-confidence/some social integration/makes some decisions and influences control in familiar situations.

3 Some self-confidence; autonomy emerging. Makes decisions and has control of some aspects of life. Able to achieve some limited social integration/educational activities. Diffident over control over life. Needs encouragement to achieve potential.

4 Mostly confident; occasional difficulties integrating or in fulfilling social/role activity. Participates in all appropriate decisions. May have difficulty in achieving potential in some situations occasionally.

5 Achieving potential. Autonomous and unrestricted. Able to fulfil social, educational and family role.

Wellbeing/Distress (client/carer)

0 Severe constant: Upset/frustration/anger/distress/embarrassment/concern/withdrawal. High and constant levels of concern/anger/severe depression/apathy. Unable to express or control emotions appropriately.

1 Frequently severe: Upset/frustration/anger/distress/embarrassment/concern/withdrawal. Moderate concern, becomes concerned easily, requires constant reassurance/support, needs clear/tight limits and structure, loses emotional control easily.

2 Moderate consistent: Upset/frustration/anger/distress/embarrassment/concern/withdrawal. Concern in unfamiliar situation, frequent emotional encouragement and support required.

3 Moderate frequent: Upset/frustration/anger/distress/embarrassment/concern/withdrawal. Controls emotions with assistance, emotionally dependent on some occasions, vulnerable to change in routine, etc., spontaneously uses methods to assist emotional control.

4 Mild occasional: Upset/frustration/anger/distress/embarrassment/concern/withdrawal. Able to control feelings in most situations, generally well adjusted/stable (most of the time/most situations), occasional emotional support/encouragement needed.

5 Not inappropriate: Upset/frustration/anger/distress/embarrassment/concern/withdrawal/severe depression/apathy.

35 Mental Health: Anxiety Disorders

Identify descriptor that is 'best fit'. The patient/client/student does not have to have each feature mentioned. Use 0.5 to indicate if patient/client/student is slightly better or worse than a descriptor and as appropriate to age.

Impairment

0 Profound. Continual demonstration of global severe symptoms with no relief.

1 Severe anxiety/stress symptoms demonstrated most of the time but occasionally, in some situations, partial relief is experienced.

2 Some situations/times when anxiety/stress is severe or moderate anxiety/stress frequently experienced (daily) but there are periods when anxiety is not a problem.

3 Anxiety/stress occasionally severe (weekly) can manage stress on some occasions but may need prompting and support with strategies.

4 Anxiety/stress levels easily aroused but copes when strategies in place, very occasional difficulties.

5 Normal response in stressful situations.

Activity

0 Physically dependent for all functional tasks. No self-care skills.

1 Dependent for most tasks but will cooperate. Physical assistance, encouragement and support required frequently. Carer undertakes burden of tasks.

2 Needs verbal and physical prompts to initiate most tasks.

3 Some physical/verbal support and encouragement to complete some tasks but initiates appropriately.

4 Occasional verbal encouragement needed and support or extra time required for specific tasks.

5 Independent in all areas.

Participation

0 Unable to fulfil any social/educational/family role. Not involved in decision making/ no autonomy/no control over environment, no social integration.

1 Low self-confidence/poor self-esteem/limited social integration/socially isolated/ contributes to some basic and limited decisions. Cannot achieve potential in any situation.

2 Some self-confidence/some social integration/makes some decisions and influences control in familiar situations.

3 Some self-confidence; autonomy emerging. Makes decisions and has control of some aspects of life. Able to achieve some limited social integration/educational activities. Diffident over control over life. Needs encouragement to achieve potential.

4 Mostly confident; occasional difficulties integrating or in fulfilling social/role activity. Participates in all appropriate decisions. May have difficulty in achieving potential in some situations occasionally.

5 Achieving potential. Autonomous and unrestricted. Able to fulfil social, educational and family role.

Wellbeing/Distress (client/carer)

0 Severe constant: Upset/frustration/anger/distress/embarrassment/concern/withdrawal. High and constant levels of concern/anger/severe depression/apathy. Unable to express or control emotions appropriately.

1 Frequently severe: Upset/frustration/anger/distress/embarrassment/concern/ withdrawal. Moderate concern, becomes concerned easily, requires constant reassurance/ support, needs clear/tight limits and structure, loses emotional control easily.

2 Moderate consistent: Upset/frustration/anger/distress/embarrassment/concern/ withdrawal. Concern in unfamiliar situation, frequent emotional encouragement and support required.

3 Moderate frequent: Upset/frustration/anger/distress/embarrassment/concern/ withdrawal. Controls emotions with assistance, emotionally dependent on some occasions, vulnerable to change in routine, etc., spontaneously uses methods to assist emotional control.

4 Mild occasional: Upset/frustration/anger/distress/embarrassment/concern/withdrawal. Able to control feelings in most situations, generally well adjusted/stable (most of the time/most situations), occasional emotional support/encouragement needed.

5 Not inappropriate: Upset/frustration/anger/distress/embarrassment/concern/ withdrawal, severe depression/apathy.

36 Multifactorial Conditions

Includes complex physical disability and frail elderly. Identify descriptor that is 'best fit'. The patient/client/student does not have to have each feature mentioned. Use 0.5 to indicate if patient/client/student is slightly better or worse than a descriptor and as appropriate to age.

Impairment

0 Profound. Inability to respond to external stimuli/gross loss of passive range of movement affecting multiple joints. Debilitated, minimal muscle power, multi-joint contractures/swelling. Total flaccidity/severe spasticity. Severe continual involuntary movements. Total loss of righting and equilibrium reactions. Global severity of all symptoms.

1 Responsive but uncooperative, range of movement maximally restricted, multiple joint involvement. Passive range of movement moderately restricted. Pain on passive movement. No standing balance. Unable to weight bear. Minimal voluntary movement. Severe sensory inattention. Low tone/moderate spasticity. Strong associated reactions. Severe degree of several signs and symptoms, for example, dense hemiplegia with some perceptual deficit. Responsive.

2 Aware and some cooperation. Active range of movement moderately restricted. Contractures in more than one joint. Pain on active movement. Poor static balance. Occasional purposeful movement. Moderate to severe inattention. Moderate involuntary movement. Associated reactions occurring on preparation to movement.

3 Aware and actively cooperative. Some active contribution to activities, active functional range of movement with minimal restriction. Intermittent pain on active movement. Poor dynamic standing balance, at risk of contractions. Some associated reactions during movement. Purposeful but not necessarily accurate voluntary movement. Moderate sensory inattention. Minimal involuntary movement. May have one severe sign or symptom alone, for example dense hemiplegia or severe perceptual deficit or a combination of milder signs or symptoms, for example mild hemiparesis with some sensory loss.

4 Cooperative, may have mild occasional inattention. Slight/minimal abnormality of strength, muscle tone, range of movement. Occasional difficulty with balance, purposeful accurate voluntary movements. May have abnormal speed of movement, slight incoordination. Minimal associated reaction with efforts.

5 Age-appropriate strength, range of movement and coordination. Normal tone and active movements.

Activity

0 No purposeful active movement, totally dependent, requires full physical care and constant vigilant supervision. May have totally disruptive and uncooperative behaviour. Dependent on skilled assistance.

1 Bed/chair-bound but unable to sit independently. Some very limited purposeful activity. Needs high level of assistance in most tasks. Some awareness, some effort and recognition to contribute to care. Dependent on skilled assistance.

2 Head and trunk control. Limited self-help skills. Initiates some aspects of ADL. Transfers with one, mobilizes with two. Requires physical and verbal prompting and supervision for most tasks and movements. Partakes in care and engages in some structured activity. Dependent on skilled assistance.

3 Transfers or walking requires supervision or help of one. Undertakes personal care in modified supported environment. Needs assistance or supervision with some unfamiliar or complex tasks. Initiates activities appropriately.

4 Carries out personal care and tasks but is less efficient, clumsy, requires extra time or may need encouragement. Uses memory prompts effectively. Minimal or occasional assistance required for some complex tasks.

5 Age-appropriate independence.

Participation

0 Unable to fulfil any social/educational/family role. Not involved in decision making/ no autonomy/no control over environment, no social integration.

1 Low self-confidence/poor self-esteem/limited social integration/socially isolated/ contributes to some basic and limited decisions. Cannot achieve potential in any situation.

2 Some self-confidence/some social integration/makes some decisions and influences control in familiar situations.

3 Some self-confidence; autonomy emerging. Makes decisions and has control of some aspects of life. Able to achieve some limited social integration/educational activities. Diffident over control over life. Needs encouragement to achieve potential.

4 Mostly confident; occasional difficulties integrating or in fulfilling social/role activity. Participates in all appropriate decisions. May have difficulty in achieving potential in some situations occasionally.

5 Achieving potential. Autonomous and unrestricted. Able to fulfil social, educational and family role.

Wellbeing/Distress (client/carer)

0 Severe constant: High and constant levels of distress/upset/concern/frustration/ anger/embarrassment/withdrawal/severe depression/apathy. Unable to express or control emotions appropriately.

1 Frequently severe: Moderate distress/upset/concern/frustration/anger/embarrassment/ withdrawal/severe depression/apathy. Becomes concerned easily, requires constant reassurance/support, needs clear/tight limits and structure, loses emotional control easily.

2 Moderate consistent: Distress/upset/concern/frustration/anger/embarrassment/ withdrawal/severe depression/apathy in unfamiliar situations, frequent emotional encouragement and support required.

3 Moderate frequent: Distress/upset/concern/frustration/anger/embarrassment/ withdrawal/severe depression/apathy. Controls emotions with assistance, emotionally dependent on some occasions, vulnerable to change in routine, etc., spontaneously uses methods to assist emotional control.

4 Mild occasional: Distress/upset/concern/frustration/anger/embarrassment/withdrawal/ severe depression/apathy. Able to control feelings in most situations, generally well adjusted/stable (most of the time/most situations), occasional emotional support/ encouragement needed.

5 Not inappropriate: Distress/upset/concern/frustration/anger/embarrassment/ withdrawal/severe depression/apathy. Well adjusted, stable and able to cope emotionally with most situations, good insight, accepts and understands own limitations.

37 Musculoskeletal

Identify descriptor that is 'best fit'. The patient/client/student does not have to have each feature mentioned. Use 0.5 to indicate if patient/client/student is slightly better or worse than a descriptor and as appropriate to age.

Impairment

0 Profound. Crippling, chronic, severe non-reversible deformity, severe inhibiting pain in several joints/parts of body. Severely limited range of movement and muscle power.

1 Severely restricted range of movement, partially reversible deformity, constant inhibiting pain/abnormal tone.

2 Moderate reversible deformity, restricted range of movement, redeemable muscle damage, inhibiting pain causing altered movement, moderate increased or decreased muscle tone. Poor exercise tolerance.

3 Correctable/slight deformity/slight increase or decrease in muscle tone, 60% range of movement and muscle power. Intermittent pain resulting in occasional altered practice. Some inhibiting pain. Moderate exercise tolerance.

4 Slightly reduced muscle power, 80% range of movement, good exercise tolerance. Occasional discomfort.

5 Full range of movement and power. No pain, no abnormal muscle tone.

Activity

0 Immobile, totally dependent in all/any environments. Unable to participate in tasks.

1 Can transfer with maximal skilled physical assistance. Requires maximal assistance with all personal activities of daily living.

2 Requires regular assistance with activities of daily living, can undertake some tasks independently.

3 Personal activities of daily living/transfers requiring supervision and some occasional help from carer.

4 Independent in adapted environment, needs occasional assistance or extra time with complex or unfamiliar activities.

5 Age-appropriate independence in all environments.

Participation

0 Unable to fulfil any social/educational/family role. Not involved in decision making/ no autonomy/no control over environment, no social integration.

1 Low self-confidence/poor self-esteem/limited social integration/socially isolated/ contributes to some basic and limited decisions. Cannot achieve potential in any situation.

2 Some self-confidence/some social integration/makes some decisions and influences control in familiar situations.

3 Some self-confidence; autonomy emerging. Makes decisions and has control of some aspects of life. Able to achieve some limited social integration/educational activities. Diffident over control over life. Needs encouragement to achieve potential.

4 Mostly confident; occasional difficulties integrating or in fulfilling social/role activity. Participates in all appropriate decisions. May have difficulty in achieving potential in some situations occasionally.

5 Achieving potential. Autonomous and unrestricted. Able to fulfil social, educational and family role.

Wellbeing/Distress (client/carer)

0 Severe constant: Upset/frustration/anger/distress/embarrassment/concern/withdrawal. High and constant levels of concern/anger/severe depression/apathy. Unable to express or control emotions appropriately.

1 Frequently severe: Upset/frustration/anger/distress/embarrassment/concern/ withdrawal. Moderate concern, becomes concerned easily, requires constant reassurance/ support, needs clear/tight limits and structure, loses emotional control easily.

2 Moderate consistent: Upset/frustration/anger/distress/embarrassment/concern/ withdrawal. Concern in unfamiliar situation, frequent emotional encouragement and support required.

3 Moderate frequent: Upset/frustration/anger/distress/embarrassment/concern/ withdrawal. Controls emotions with assistance, emotionally dependent on some occasions, vulnerable to change in routine, etc., spontaneously uses methods to assist emotional control.

4 Mild occasional: Upset/frustration/anger/distress/embarrassment/concern/withdrawal. Able to control feelings in most situations, generally well adjusted/stable (most of the time/most situations), occasional emotional support/encouragement needed.

5 Not inappropriate: Upset/frustration/anger/distress/embarrassment/concern/ withdrawal.

38 Neurological Disorders (including Progressive Neurological Disorders)

Identify descriptor that is 'best fit'. The patient/client/student does not have to have each feature mentioned. Use 0.5 to indicate if patient/client/student is slightly better or worse than a descriptor and as appropriate to age.

Impairment

0 Profound. No volitional movement. Total flaccidity/severe spasticity. Total sensory inattention. Severe continual involuntary movement. Total loss of righting plus equilibrium reactions. Severe global symptoms. May be primarily bedbound.

1 Occasional minimal voluntary movements. Severe loss of motor or sensory function, with severe flaccidity/spasticity. All limbs and trunk affected. Moderate to severe involuntary movements. Severe sensory inattention.

2 Frequent voluntary movements. Moderate involuntary movement. General associated reactions occurring on preparation to movement. Moderate to severe inattention.

3 Minimal involuntary movements. Severe abnormal tone in specific muscle groups or moderate impairment of tone globally. Specific associated reactions during preparation to move. Purposeful and controlled but not necessarily accurate or strong voluntary movement. Moderate sensory inattention.

4 Mild abnormality of tone or minimal or occasional associated reactions with effort. Can control tone but occasional abnormal tone, for example after activity. Purposeful accurate voluntary movement. Abnormal speed of movement. Minimal sensory inattention.

5 Normal purposeful skilled movement. Normal tone, normal sensory awareness, normal righting and equilibrium reactions, alert and orientated.

Activity

0 No purposeful active movement, totally dependent, requires full physical care and constant vigilant supervision. May have totally disruptive and uncooperative behaviour. Dependent on skilled assistance.

1 Bed/chair-bound but poor trunk control. Transfers with maximal assistance, wheelchair dependent, unable to stand unsupported. Some very limited purposeful activity. Needs high level of assistance in all tasks. Some awareness, some effort and recognition to contribute to care. Dependent on skilled assistance.

2 Head and trunk control. Limited self-help skills but initiates some aspects of ADL. Transfers with one, mobilizes with two. Requires physical and/or verbal prompting and supervision for most tasks and movements. Participates in care and engaging in some structured activity. Dependent on skilled assistance.

3 Stands unsupported, transfers or walking requires supervision or help of one. 'House hold walker'. Undertakes personal care in modified supported environment. Needs assistance or supervision with some unfamiliar or complex tasks. Initiates activities appropriately. Ability varies with time of day.

4 Carries out personal care and tasks but is less efficient, clumsy, requires extra time or may need encouragement. Uses prompts effectively. Minimal or occasional assistance required for some complex tasks.

5 Age-appropriate independence.

Participation

0 Unable to fulfil any social/educational/family role. Not involved in decision making/ no autonomy/no control over environment, no social integration.

1 Low self-confidence/poor self-esteem/limited social integration/socially isolated/ contributes to some basic and limited decisions. Cannot achieve potential in any situation.

2 Some self-confidence/some social integration/makes some decisions and influences control in familiar situations.

3 Some self-confidence; autonomy emerging. Makes decisions and has control of some aspects of life. Able to achieve some limited social integration/educational activities. Diffident over control over life. Needs encouragement to achieve potential.

4 Mostly confident; occasional difficulties integrating or in fulfilling social/role activity. Participates in all appropriate decisions. May have difficulty in achieving potential in some situations occasionally.

5 Achieving potential. Autonomous and unrestricted. Able to fulfil social, educational and family role.

Wellbeing/Distress (client/carer)

0 Severe constant: High and constant levels of distress/upset/concern/frustration/ anger/embarrassment/withdrawal/severe depression/apathy. Unable to express or control emotions appropriately.

1 Frequently severe: Moderate distress/upset/concern/frustration/anger/embarrassment/ withdrawal/severe depression/apathy. Becomes concerned easily, requires constant reassurance/support, needs clear/tight limits and structure, loses emotional control easily.

2 Moderate consistent: Distress/upset/concern/frustration/anger/embarrassment/ withdrawal/severe depression/apathy in unfamiliar situations. Frequent emotional encouragement and support required.

3 Moderate frequent: Distress/upset/concern/frustration/anger/embarrassment/ withdrawal/severe depression/apathy. Controls emotions with assistance, emotionally dependent on some occasions, vulnerable to change in routine, etc., spontaneously uses methods to assist emotional control.

4 Mild occasional: Distress/upset/concern/frustration/anger/embarrassment/withdrawal/ severe depression/apathy. Able to control feelings in most situations, generally well adjusted/stable (most of the time/most situations), occasional emotional support/ encouragement needed.

5 Not inappropriate: Distress/upset/concern/frustration/anger/embarrassment/ withdrawal/severe depression/apathy. Well adjusted, stable and able to cope emotionally with most situations, good insight, accepts and understands own limitations.

39 Palliative Care

Identify descriptor that is 'best fit'. The patient/client/student does not have to have each feature mentioned. Use 0.5 to indicate if patient/client/student is slightly better or worse than a descriptor and as appropriate to age.

Impairment

0 Profound. Severe, constant symptom burden, for example pain/weakness in multiple sites; severe constant breathlessness/fatigue/nausea/impaired cognition. Symptoms not relieved by medication or non-pharmacological methods.

1 Constant moderate and intermittently severe episodes of symptom burden. For example, moderate/intermittently severe pain/weakness in two or more sites; moderate/intermittently severe breathlessness/fatigue/nausea/impaired cognition. Little reduction in symptoms with medication or non-pharmacological methods.

2 Constant moderate levels of symptom burden. For example, constant moderate pain/weakness in one or more sites; constant moderate breathlessness/fatigue/nausea/impaired cognition. Frequent, intermittent relief from medication or other non-pharmacological methods.

3 Moderate/ intermittently mild symptom burden. Periods of pain/weakness/breathlessness/fatigue/nausea/impaired cognition. Some improvement from medication or non-pharmacological methods.

4 Intermittent or mild symptom burden. Pain/weakness/breathlessness/fatigue/nausea/impaired cognition. Symptoms are mostly relieved with medication and/or non-pharmacological methods such as personal strategies.

5 No symptom burden.

Activity

0 No purposeful active movement, totally dependent, requires full physical care and constant vigilant supervision. Totally dependent on skilled assistance.

1 Some very limited purposeful activity. Bed/chair-bound, unable to sit independently. Needs high level of assistance in most tasks. Some awareness, some effort and recognition to contribute to care. Dependent on skilled assistance.

2 Participates in care and engages in some structured activity. Limited self-help skills. Initiates some aspects of activities of daily living (ADL). Transfers with one, mobilizes with two. Requires physical and verbal prompting and supervision for most tasks and movements. Dependent on familiar assistance.

3 Appropriately initiates activities. Transfers or walking requires help or supervision of one. Undertakes personal care in a modified supported environment. Needs assistance or supervision with some unfamiliar or complex tasks.

4 Independent in familiar and/or adapted environments. Carries out personal care and other activities of daily living but is less efficient. Needs occasional assistance and/or extra time with physically demanding activities.

5 Activity not restricted.

Participation

0 Unable to fulfil any meaningful and/or purposeful role. Unable to participate in any decision making. No social integration. No future plans in place and unable to take part in decision making about the future.

1 Requires full, skilled assistance to participate in any purposeful and/or meaningful role. Contributes to some basic and limited decision making. Unable to initiate social integration, low self-confidence/poor self-esteem and socially withdrawn. Can make simple choices but unable to contribute to complex future planning.

2 Some participation in familiar purposeful or meaningful roles. Able to engage more readily in some limited social integration. Able to respond to some social integration and some self-confidence but requires support (physical and/or emotional). Able to express preferences spontaneously for future care but requires support to weigh up options, plan and implement.

3 Able to recognize and appropriately participate in purposeful and meaningful roles. Able to make some decisions and understands potential consequences. Able to seek out and respond to social integration of their own choice but needs physical and/or emotional support. Some self-confidence, and able to contribute to future planning.

4 Occasional difficulty in fulfilling purposeful or meaningful roles. Able to seek out and respond to social integration of their choice. Minor restrictions in some situations but mostly confident; participates in all appropriate decisions and future planning.

5 Able to fulfil purposeful and meaningful roles. Autonomous decision making and social integration. Support in future planning for complex issues only.

Wellbeing/Distress (client/carer)

0 Severe, constant levels of distress: High and constant levels of distress/concern/anxiety/fear/grief/boredom. Unable to express or control emotions appropriately. No enjoyment of any activities. Unable to adjust to situation. No effective coping mechanism/strategy.

1 Frequently severe levels of distress: Frequent and significant levels of distress/concern/anxiety/fear/grief/boredom. Infrequent signs of pleasure or enjoyment. Loses emotional control easily. Shows some signs of adjustment but much difficulty with this. Coping mechanisms are frequently ineffective.

2 Moderate consistent levels of distress: Signs of distress/concern/anxiety/fear/grief/boredom in unfamiliar situations. Signs of pleasure or enjoyment in familiar situations/activities. Frequent emotional encouragement and support is required. Difficulty with adjustment; requires support. Coping mechanisms used with support and some success.

3 Moderate frequent levels of distress: Some signs of distress/concern/anxiety/fear/grief/boredom. Is able to control emotions with assistance but is vulnerable to change in routine. Spontaneously uses methods to assist emotional controls in familiar situations. Very occasionally has difficulty enjoying activities. Well adjusted most of the time but occasionally requiring support. Unable to cope with some aspects of condition.

4 Mild, occasional levels of distress: Occasional signs of distress/concern/anxiety/fear/grief/boredom. Able to control feelings in most situations, generally well adjusted/stable (most of the time/most situations), occasional emotional support/encouragement needed. Frequent and consistent signs of pleasure and enjoyment. Copes well most of the time, uses strategies effectively.

5 Not inappropriate levels of distress: Generally well adjusted. Appropriate enjoyment of activities. Stable and able to cope emotionally with most situations, good insight into own limitations.

40 Phonological Disorder

The individual does not have to have each feature mentioned in the descriptor. It is a best fit description, i.e., does this description fit the individual better than the other one. Use 0.5 to indicate if the individual is slightly better or worse than the descriptor. Consider as appropriate for age.

Impairment*

0 Profound. No phonological system; limited range of sounds used.

1 Severe – four or more inappropriate phonological processes for the child's age; more than 80% inconsistency rating. More than two elements of disorder, e.g., sounds, substitutions, omissions.

2 Severe/moderate – three inappropriate phonological processes for the child's age; 60–80% inconsistency rating. Two elements of disorder, e.g., sounds, substitutions, omissions.

3 Moderate – two inappropriate phonological processes for the child's age; 40–60% inconsistency rating. One element of disorder, e.g., sounds, substitutions, omissions.

4 Mild – one inappropriate phonological process for the child's age; 40% inconsistency rating.

5 Age-appropriate speech.

Activity

0 Completely unintelligible to familiar and non-familiar listeners.

1 Partly intelligible to familiar listeners in known context; communication partner bears the burden of the responsibility.

2 Intelligible to familiar listeners in context; partly intelligible in context with non-familiar listeners; unintelligible in connected speech.

3 Usually intelligible to familiar listeners in and out of context; variable intelligibility in context with non-familiar listeners; free, spontaneous speech can be unintelligible.

4 Minor problems evident but intelligible to everyone; occasionally loses intelligibility, for example when excited or speaking against noise, etc.

5 Intelligible at age-appropriate level to familiar listeners and non-familiar listeners.

Participation

0 Unable to fulfil any social/educational/family role. Not involved in decision-making, no autonomy, no control over environment, no social integration.

1 Low self-confidence, poor self-esteem, limited social integration, socially isolated, contributes to some basic and limited decisions. Cannot achieve potential in any situation.

2 Some self-confidence, some social integration, makes some decisions and influences control in familiar situations.

3 Some self-confidence; autonomy emerging. Makes decisions and has control of some aspects of life. Able to achieve some limited social integration/educational activities. Diffident over control over life. Needs encouragement to achieve potential.

4 Mostly confident. Occasional difficulties in integrating or in fulfilling social/role activity. Participates in all appropriate decisions. May have difficulty in achieving potential in some situations occasionally.

5 Achieving potential. Autonomous and unrestricted. Able to fulfil social, educational and family role.

Wellbeing/Distress (client/carer)

0 Severe constant: High and constant levels of distress/upset/concern/frustration/anger/embarrassment/withdrawal/severe depression/apathy. Unable to express or control emotions appropriately.

1 Frequently severe: Moderate distress/upset/concern/frustration/anger/embarrassment/withdrawal/severe depression/apathy. Becomes concerned easily, requires constant reassurance/support, needs clear/tight limits and structure, loses emotional control easily.

2 Moderate consistent: Distress/upset/concern/frustration/anger/embarrassment/withdrawal/severe depression/apathy in unfamiliar situations. Frequent emotional encouragement and support required.

3 Moderate frequent: Distress/upset/concern/frustration/anger/embarrassment/withdrawal/severe depression/apathy. Controls emotions with assistance, emotionally dependent on some occasions, vulnerable to change in routine, etc., spontaneously uses methods to assist emotional control.

4 Mild occasional: Distress/upset/concern/frustration/anger/embarrassment/withdrawal/severe depression/apathy. Able to control feelings in most situations, generally well adjusted/stable (most of the time/most situations), occasional emotional support/encouragement needed.

5 Not inappropriate: Distress/upset/concern/frustration/anger/embarrassment/withdrawal/severe depression/apathy. Well adjusted, stable and able to cope emotionally with most situations, good insight, accepts and understands own limitations.

*Impairment based on: Barbara Dodd, Zhu Hua, Sharon Crosbie, Alison Holm, Anne Ozanne (2002). *Diagnostic Evaluation of Articulation and Phonology* (DEAP). London: Pearson.

Acknowledgement: Developed by Rachel Brown and Nicola Cuthbert-Brown (Surrey County Council SLT Service)

41 Podiatric Conditions

Identify descriptor that is 'best fit'. The patient/client/student does not have to have each feature mentioned. Use 0.5 to indicate if patient/client/student is slightly better or worse than a descriptor and as appropriate to age.

Impairment

0 Profound podiatric condition. Gangrene. Necrosis. Acute ischaemia, septicaemia. Generalized infection. Perforated ulcer. Malignancy. Osteomyelitis. Category 3/4 or unstageable ulcer with generalized infection. Severe pain (9/10) in foot not relieved by medication. Recurrent continual podiatric conditions requiring intensive professional attention.

1 Severe podiatric condition. Severe infection. Gross deformity. Dislocation. Peripheral neuropathy. Severe localized infection. Category 4 ulcer with infection or osteomyelitis. Nail condition with local cellulitis. Severe callus/corn with extravasation or breakdown. Severe pain in foot (7/8), some relief with strong medication. Recurrent continual podiatric conditions requiring intensive professional attention.

2 Severe/moderate podiatric condition. High risk of ulceration/Category 3 ulcer. Infection in nail. Inflammation. Continual complications, e.g., sinus complicated by mechanical problem. Severe callus/corn formation. Severe pain (5/6) relieved by strong medication. Recurrent continual podiatric conditions requiring regular professional attention.

3 Moderate podiatric condition. Corns/callus/tinea which are problematical. Involuted nails. Non-infective O/C. Nail pathologies, nail plate destruction, heel pain, dermal fissures uncomplicated by mechanical problem. Moderate pain (3/4) relieved with medication or other strategies. Recurrent continual podiatric conditions requiring regular professional attention.

4 Mild podiatric condition. Risk of ulceration. Mild or occasional pain in foot (1/2), minor mechanical problem. Non-painful nail pathology. Minor skin/nail condition requiring attention or advice.

5 No podiatric condition. Normal functioning feet. Normal skin and nails.

Activity

0 Bed-bound or no mobility because of unremitting pain. Sleep continually disturbed. All activities inhibited. Unable to function independently. Unable to tolerate footwear.

1 Severely restricted mobility. Requires heavy support for any movement. Assistance required for all activities. Able to tolerate adapted footwear for short periods.

2 Mobility restricted to around the house. Can weight bear but in continual discomfort leading to restlessness, needs substantial assistance for all activities. Able to tolerate adapted footwear.

3 Intermittent pain restricting activity, unable to walk or stand for long periods of time. Limitations on mobility affecting daily activities. Can wear normal footwear for short periods of time.

4 Activity is only occasionally restricted, prefers certain range of footwear for comfort. Minor and occasional limitation on mobility.

5 No restriction on activity, mobility or footwear.

Participation

0 No autonomy, isolated. Not able to engage in work, school or social activities.

1 Very limited choices, severe limitations on work, school and social activities, little control over life.

2 Some integration, value and autonomy in one setting. Work, school and social activities severely restricted.

3 Integrated, valued and autonomous in limited number of settings. Work, school and social activities restricted to short periods of time or require special adaptations/support.

4 Occasionally some restriction in autonomy, integration or role. Occasional restriction with work, school or social activities.

5 Integrated, valued, occupies appropriate role, unrestricted engagement.

Wellbeing/Distress (client/carer)

0 Severe constant: High and constant levels of distress/upset/concern/frustration/anger/embarrassment/withdrawal/severe depression/apathy. Unable to express or control emotions appropriately.

1 Frequently severe: Moderate distress/upset/concern/frustration/anger/embarrassment/withdrawal/severe depression/apathy. Becomes concerned easily, requires constant reassurance/support, needs clear/tight limits and structure, loses emotional control easily.

2 Moderate consistent: Distress/upset/concern/frustration/anger/embarrassment/withdrawal/severe depression/apathy in unfamiliar situations, frequent emotional encouragement and support required.

3 Moderate frequent: Distress/upset/concern/frustration/anger/embarrassment/withdrawal/severe depression/apathy. Controls emotions with assistance, emotionally dependent on some occasions, vulnerable to change in routine, etc., spontaneously uses methods to assist emotional control.

4 Mild occasional: Distress/upset/concern/frustration/anger/embarrassment/withdrawal/severe depression/apathy. Able to control feelings in most situations, generally well adjusted/stable (most of the time/most situations), occasional emotional support/encouragement needed.

5 Not inappropriate: Distress/upset/concern/frustration/anger/embarrassment/withdrawal/severe depression/apathy. Well adjusted, stable and able to cope emotionally with most situations, good insight, accepts and understands own limitations.

42 Postnatal Depression

Identify descriptor that is 'best fit'. The patient/client/student does not have to have each feature mentioned. Use 0.5 to indicate if patient/client/student is slightly better or worse than a descriptor and as appropriate to age.

Impairment

0 Catatonic, persistent and severe low mood with no relief, no interest or engagement in activities, unable to experience pleasure from all activities usually found enjoyable and no motivation. Psychomotor retardation or agitation most days. May include psychotic symptoms, e.g., delusions/hallucinations.

1 Persistent and severe low mood with very occasional relief. Intense feelings of guilt. Delusions and/or fixed negative beliefs including frequent thoughts of harming the baby and/or self. Unable to experience pleasure from most activities usually found enjoyable. Inability to make decisions. Extreme lack of energy.

2 Severe low mood, feeling depressed most of the time, experiences only occasional pleasure, occasional relief from symptoms. Some thoughts of death, suicide and/or harming the baby. Unable to experience pleasure from several activities usually found enjoyable Frequent negative beliefs that may respond to reassurance. Reduced energy, fatigue most days.

3 Moderate low mood, frequently feeling depressed but gains some pleasure from certain activities and with the baby. Infrequent thoughts of death and/or harming the baby. Unable to experience pleasure from a few activities usually found enjoyable. Some energy, unusual fatigue some of the time.

4 Occasional, mild low mood, occasional problems with motivation, decision making and concentration. Experiences pleasure from most activities usually found enjoyable. Mood reactive to circumstances, may be more vulnerable to stress than usual, uses strategies to cope.

5 No persistent low mood or anhedonia, normal responses to stressful situations.

Activity

0 Dependent on others for self-care and all other activities of daily living. Unable to provide care for the baby or respond to the baby's cues/no interaction with baby.

1 High level of support and assistance in all self-care and high level of support to recognize baby's needs and respond to them, minimal interaction with baby.

2 Able to cooperate in self-care with support and prompting. Able to recognize baby's needs with support to meet them. Some interaction with baby.

3 Initiating self-care. Needs prompting on some occasions to initiate care for baby. Responds to cues, able to have some independence with regular support and encouragement. Independent in familiar surroundings.

4 Able to live independently with some occasional support. Assistance and support may be required in unfamiliar surroundings.

5 Fully independent. Caring for baby and self appropriately.

Participation

0 Unable to fulfil any social/educational/family role. Not involved in decision making/ no autonomy/no control over environment, no social integration.

1 Low self-confidence/poor self-esteem/limited social integration/socially isolated/ contributes to basic and limited decisions. Cannot achieve potential in any situation.

2 Some self-confidence/some social integration/makes some decisions and influences control in familiar situations.

3 Some self-confidence; autonomy emerging. Makes decisions and has some control of some aspects of life. Able to achieve some limited social integration/educational activities. Diffident over control over life. Needs encouragement to achieve potential.

4 Mostly confident: Occasional difficulties integrating or fulfilling social/role activity. Participates in all relevant decisions. May have difficulty in achieving potential in some situations occasionally.

5 Achieving potential. Autonomous and unrestricted. Able to fulfil social, educational and family role

Wellbeing/distress

0 Severe constant: Frustration/guilt/anger/distress/worthless/embarrassment/concern/ withdrawal. High and constant levels of concern/anger/severe depression/apathy. Unable to express or control emotions appropriately.

1 Frequent severe: Frustration/guilt/anger/distress/worthless/embarrassment/concern/ withdrawal. Moderate concern, becomes concerned easily, requires constant reassurance/ support, needs clear/tight limits and structure, loses emotional control easily.

2 Moderate consistent: Frustration/guilt/anger/distress/worthless/embarrassment/ concern/withdrawal. Concern in unfamiliar situations, frequent emotional encouragement and support required.

3 Moderate frequent: Frustration/guilt/anger/distress/worthless/embarrassment/concern/withdrawal. Controls emotions with assistance, emotionally dependent on some occasions, vulnerable to change in routine, etc., spontaneously uses methods to assist emotional control.

4 Mild occasional: Frustration/guilt/anger/distress/worthless/embarrassment/concern/withdrawal. Able to control feelings in most situations, generally well adjusted/stable (most of the time/most situations), occasional emotional support/encouragement needed.

5 Not inappropriate: Frustration/guilt/anger/distress/worthless/embarrassment/concern/withdrawal.

43 Respiratory Care:
Chronic Obstructive Pulmonary Disease (COPD)

Identify descriptor that is 'best fit'. The patient/client/student does not have to have each feature mentioned. Use 0.5 to indicate if patient/client/student is slightly better or worse than a descriptor and as appropriate to age.

Impairment

0 Profound. Full ventilatory support.

1 Some ventilatory support required, for example, at night. Retains secretions/airway obstruction or altered air blood gases.

2 Requires regular oxygen therapy/medication. Altered use of respiratory muscles. Help required to clear secretions. Altered air blood gases.

3 Lung function maintained with regular medication. Frequently normal air blood gases. Frequent productive cough, occasional problem with self-clearing of secretions.

4 Normal lung function maintained with minimum medication. Non-problematic self-clearing of secretions. Normal air blood gases.

5 Normal lung function.

Activity

0 Unable to move, breathlessness at rest. Total care required (room-bound).

1 Severe breathlessness on movement in bed, severe orthopnea, breathlessness affecting fluency of speech, requires maximal help in all activities (house-bound).

2 Severe breathlessness on minimal exertion, i.e., transfer from bed to chair, any effort affects speech. Can undertake a few ADL tasks unaided (house/immediate environment-bound).

3 Breathlessness walking on level ground (50 yards). Normal speech when undertaking light activity. Independent for limited activities (access to local environment).

4 Breathlessness on flight of stairs, not breathless on level ground. Occasional reduction in complex or demanding tasks due to pain/breathlessness.

5 No functional disability, able to tackle exertion appropriate to age without respiratory distress.

Participation

0 Unable to fulfil any social/educational/family role. Not involved in decision making/ no autonomy/no control over environment; no social integration.

1 Low self-confidence/poor self-esteem/limited social integration/socially isolated/ contributes to some basic and limited decisions. Cannot achieve potential in any situation.

2 Some self-confidence/some social integration/makes some decisions and influences control in familiar situations.

3 Some self-confidence; autonomy emerging. Makes decisions and has control of some aspects of life. Able to achieve some limited social integration/educational activities. Diffident over control over life. Needs encouragement to achieve potential.

4 Mostly confident; occasional difficulties integrating or in fulfilling social/role activity. Participates in all appropriate decisions. May have difficulty in achieving potential in some situations occasionally.

5 Achieving potential. Autonomous and unrestricted. Able to fulfil social, educational and family role.

Wellbeing/Distress (client/carer)

0 Severe constant: Upset/frustration/anger/distress/embarrassment/concern/withdrawal. High and constant levels of concern/anger/severe depression/apathy. Unable to express or control emotions appropriately.

1 Frequently severe: Upset/frustration/anger/distress/embarrassment/concern/ withdrawal. Moderate concern, becomes concerned easily, requires constant reassurance/ support, needs clear/tight limits and structure, loses emotional control easily.

2 Moderate consistent: Upset/frustration/anger/distress/embarrassment/concern/ withdrawal. Concern in unfamiliar situation, frequent emotional encouragement and support required.

3 Moderate frequent: Upset/frustration/anger/distress/embarrassment/concern/ withdrawal. Controls emotions with assistance, emotionally dependent on some occasions, vulnerable to change in routine, etc., spontaneously uses methods to assist emotional control.

4 Mild occasional: Upset/frustration/anger/distress/embarrassment/concern/withdrawal. Able to control feelings in most situations, generally well adjusted/stable (most of the time/most situations), occasional emotional support/encouragement needed.

5 Not inappropriate: Upset/frustration/anger/distress/embarrassment/concern/ withdrawal.

44 Schizophrenia

Identify descriptor that is 'best fit'. The patient/client/student does not have to have each feature mentioned. Use 0.5 to indicate if patient/client/student is slightly better or worse than a descriptor and as appropriate to age.

Impairment

0 Profound. No insight, no volition, persistent/severe and wide range of thought disorder, fixed delusions, persistent visual, auditory, tactile hallucinations, persistent/severe disturbance of affect. Severe emotional blunting. Absence of empathy.

1 Thought disorder with variability, auditory hallucinations frequent, variable disturbance of affect, little volition. Severe-moderate emotional blunting. Very occasionally, empathy present.

2 Moderate thought disorder in duration, severity, frequency, some auditory hallucinations present, moderate disturbance of affect, moderate level of volition. Moderate emotional blunting. Empathy present to a limited extent.

3 Occasional evidence of though disorder in duration, severity, frequency, very occasional evidence of auditory hallucination, usually stable mood, volition intact. Occasional/mild emotional blunting. Appropriate empathy on occasions.

4 Very occasional evidence of some thought disorder in duration, severity, frequency, good level of insight, usually stable mood, volition intact. No emotional blunting, appropriate empathy.

5 Well-developed insight, high level of volition, no evidence of thought disorder, delusion, hallucinations, consistently stable mood.

Activity

0 Physically dependent for all functional tasks, bed/chair-bound, no self-care skills, inability to communicate, no attention.

1 Dependent for most tasks but will cooperate/assist with maximal prompting, needs cues and reminders for activities of daily living, occasional small amount of verbal communication with individual members of staff. No insight.

2 Able to initiate some aspects of activities of daily living, for example, dressing. Understandable communication increased with some meaningful content, able to concentrate for a short time, easily distracted. Needs frequent supervision and prompting. Occasional insight.

3 Some consistency in communication, for example interacting with staff/carers and other clients, able to initiate a broader range of activities of daily living, responds to demands of rehabilitation.

4 Minimal assistance needed in less familiar environments, communicating effectively with a wide range of groups and individuals, concentrating on a majority of necessary activities. Uses self-help prompts well. Good insight.

5 Independent, no assistance needed for ADL, communicating effectively with a wide range of groups and individuals, concentrates on all necessary activities.

Participation

0 Unable to fulfil any social/educational/family role. Not involved in decision making/ no autonomy/no control over environment, no social integration.

1 Low self-confidence/poor self-esteem/limited social integration/socially isolated/ contributes to some basic and limited decisions. Cannot achieve potential in any situation.

2 Some self-confidence/some social integration/makes some decisions and influences control in familiar situations.

3 Some self-confidence; autonomy emerging. Makes decisions and has control of some aspects of life. Able to achieve some limited social integration/educational activities. Diffident over control over life. Needs encouragement to achieve potential.

4 Mostly confident; occasional difficulties integrating or in fulfilling social/role activity. Participates in all appropriate decisions. May have difficulty in achieving potential in some situations occasionally.

5 Achieving potential. Autonomous and unrestricted. Able to fulfil social, educational and family role.

Wellbeing/Distress (client/carer)

0 Severe constant: Upset/frustration/anger/distress/embarrassment/concern/withdrawal. High and constant levels of concern/anger/severe depression/apathy. Unable to express or control emotions appropriately.

1 Frequently severe: Upset/frustration/anger/distress/embarrassment/concern/ withdrawal. Moderate concern, becomes concerned easily, requires constant reassurance/ support, needs clear/tight limits and structure, loses emotional control easily.

2 Moderate consistent: Upset/frustration/anger/distress/embarrassment/concern/withdrawal. Concern in unfamiliar situation, frequent emotional encouragement and support required.

3 Moderate frequent: Upset/frustration/anger/distress/embarrassment/concern/withdrawal. Controls emotions with assistance, emotionally dependent on some occasions, vulnerable to change in routine, etc., spontaneously uses methods to assist emotional control.

4 Mild occasional: Upset/frustration/anger/distress/embarrassment/concern/withdrawal. Able to control feelings in most situations, generally well adjusted/stable (most of the time/most situations), occasional emotional support/encouragement needed.

5 Not inappropriate: Upset/frustration/anger/distress/embarrassment/concern/withdrawal.

45 Stroke

Identify descriptor that is 'best fit'. The patient/client/student does not have to have each feature mentioned. Use 0.5 to indicate if patient/client/student is slightly better or worse than a descriptor and as appropriate to age.

Impairment

0 Profound. No voluntary movement, severe flaccidity or spasticity, gross sensory impairment, may have a loss of bowel and bladder control. Unresponsive.

1 Severe degree of several signs and symptoms, for example dense hemiplegia, severe perceptual deficit, occasional control of bladder and bowel, severe cognitive deficit, strong associated reactions with very limited range of passive movements. Responsive.

2 Moderate degree of several signs and symptoms, for example moderate hemiplegia and some dyspraxia, may have some bowel/bladder dysfunction. Active movement with gravity eliminated, control patterns of movement, moderate associated reactions, severe to moderate sensory deficit.

3 Active movement against gravity, controlled isolated movement, occasional associated reactions, moderate sensory inattention, movements may not be accurate, or one severe sign/symptom, for example dense hemiplegic arm, or two moderate signs/symptoms, for example moderate arm/leg hemiplegia.

4 Loss of fine active movement and coordination, minimal sensory deficit, loss of end range of movement. Slight incoordination or loss of power in limb/s, occasional perceptual cognitive or perceptual difficulties.

5 No impairment.

Activity

0 No purposeful active movement, totally dependent, requires full physical care and constant vigilant supervision. May have totally disruptive and uncooperative behaviour. Dependent on skilled assistance.

1 Bed/chair-bound but unable to sit independently. Some very limited purposeful activity. Needs high level of assistance in most tasks. Some awareness, some effort and recognition to contribute to care. Dependent on skilled assistance.

2 Head and trunk control. Limited self-help skills. Initiates some aspects of ADL. Transfers with one, mobilizes with two. Requires physical and verbal prompting and supervision for most tasks and movements. Participates in care and engages in some structured activity. Dependent on skilled assistance.

3 Transfers or walking requires supervision or help of one. Undertakes personal care in modified supported environment. Needs assistance or supervision with some unfamiliar or complex tasks. Initiates activities appropriately.

4 Carries out personal care and tasks but is less efficient, clumsy, requires extra time or may need encouragement. Uses memory prompts effectively. Minimal or occasional assistance required for some complex tasks.

5 Age-appropriate independence.

Participation

0 Unable to fulfil any social/educational/family role. Not involved in decision making/ no autonomy/no control over environment, no social integration.

1 Low self-confidence/poor self-esteem/limited social integration/socially isolated/ contributes to some basic and limited decisions. Cannot achieve potential in any situation.

2 Some self-confidence/some social integration/makes some decisions and influences control in familiar situations.

3 Some self-confidence; autonomy emerging. Makes decisions and has control of some aspects of life. Able to achieve some limited social integration/educational activities. Diffident over control over life. Needs encouragement to achieve potential.

4 Mostly confident; occasional difficulties integrating or in fulfilling social/role activity. Participates in all appropriate decisions. May have difficulty in achieving potential in some situations occasionally.

5 Achieving potential. Autonomous and unrestricted. Able to fulfil social, educational and family role.

Wellbeing/Distress (client/carer)

0 Severe constant: High and constant levels of distress/upset/concern/frustration/ anger/embarrassment/withdrawal/severe depression/apathy. Unable to express or control emotions appropriately.

1 Frequently severe: Moderate distress/upset/concern/frustration/anger/embarrassment/ withdrawal/severe depression/apathy. Becomes concerned easily, requires constant reassurance/support, needs clear/tight limits and structure, loses emotional control easily.

2 Moderate consistent: Distress/upset/concern/frustration/anger/embarrassment/ withdrawal/severe depression/apathy in unfamiliar situations. Frequent emotional encouragement and support required.

3 Moderate frequent: Distress/upset/concern/frustration/anger/embarrassment/ withdrawal/severe depression/apathy. Controls emotions with assistance, emotionally dependent on some occasions, vulnerable to change in routine, etc., spontaneously uses methods to assist emotional control.

4 Mild occasional: Distress/upset/concern/frustration/anger/embarrassment/withdrawal/ severe depression/apathy. Able to control feelings in most situations, generally well adjusted/stable (most of the time/most situations), occasional emotional support/ encouragement needed.

5 Not inappropriate: Distress/upset/concern/frustration/anger/embarrassment/ withdrawal/severe depression/apathy. Well adjusted, stable and able to cope emotionally with most situations, good insight, accepts and understands own limitations.

46 Tracheostomy

Identify descriptor that is 'best fit'. The patient/client/student does not have to have each feature mentioned. Use 0.5 to indicate if patient/client/student is slightly better or worse than a descriptor and as appropriate to age.

Impairment

0 Cuffed tracheostomy. Cuff up all the time. May have a suction aid. Requires frequent suctioning. Heavily dependent on oxygen (>4l for 24 hours). May require medication to aid secretion or respiratory management. (e.g., hyoscine/nebulizers). May require physiotherapy input.

1 Cuff partially deflated or periods of cuff deflation. Requires regular suctioning. Moderate 02 oxygen requirements (<4l for 24 hours). May require medication to aid secretion or respiratory management. May require physiotherapy input.

2 Tolerating continuous cuff deflation or cuffless tracheostomy in situ. Minimal suction and 02 required (daily but not continuous). May require medication to aid secretion or respiratory management.

3 Cuff deflated/cuffless tube. Tolerates one-way valve continuously. May require occasional suction. May require medication to aid secretion/respiratory management.

4 Cuff deflated/cuffless tube. Tolerates capping trials. Minimal/no suction required. May require medication to aid secretion/respiratory management. 4.5 decannulated. May require assistance to manage secretions (e.g., hyocine/nebulizers/oral suction).

5 Decannulated. No tracheostomy required. Stable respiratory function. Independently maintaining airway. No suction required.

Activity

0 Unable to swallow saliva or clear secretions. Unable to cough to clear secretions (including elicited). No voice. May require respiratory (O2) ventilation.

1 Sometimes able to manage secretions for short periods. Variable swallow/reduced frequency swallow. Ineffective cough. May have audible voice. May require respiratory support.

2 Able to manage secretions adequately. Effective cough. Able to swallow effectively. Audible voice attempting to use for basic communication. Minimal respiratory support.

3 Able to manage secretions independently. Tolerates increased work of breathing with a one-way valve. May be voicing with one-way valve. Able to swallow effectively. May tolerate oral intake. No additional respiratory support required (e.g., O2/ventilation).

4 Able to manage secretions independently. Tolerates increased work breathing with trials of capping. May be voicing with cap on. Able to swallow effectively. May tolerate oral intake.

5 No additional respiratory support required (e.g., O2/ventilation). No functional disability. Normal respiration and secretion management. Functional voicing. Able to maintain airway independently.

Participation

0 Unable to fulfil any social/educational/family role. Not involved in decision making/ no autonomy/no control over environment. No social integration.

1 Low self-confidence/poor self-esteem/limited social integration/socially isolated/ contributes to some basic and limited decisions. Cannot achieve potential in any situation.

2 Some self-confidence/some social integration/makes some decisions and influences control in familiar situations.

3 Some self-confidence; autonomy emerging. Makes decisions and has control of some aspects of life. Able to achieve some limited social integration/educational activities. Diffident over control over life. Needs encouragement to achieve potential.

4 Mostly confident, occasional difficulties integrating or in fulfilling social/role activity. Participates in all situations. May have difficulty in achieving potential in some situations occasionally.

5 Achieving potential, autonomous and unrestricted, Able to fulfil social, educational and family role.

Wellbeing/Distress (as appropriate to age) client/carer

0 Severe constant: Upset/frustration/anger/distress/embarrassment/concern/ withdrawal.

1 Frequently severe: Upset/frustration/anger/distress/embarrassment/concern/ withdrawal.

2 Moderate consistent: Upset/frustration/anger/distress/embarrassment/concern/ withdrawal.

3 Moderate frequent: Upset/frustration/anger/distress/embarrassment/concern/ withdrawal.

4 Mild occasional: Upset/frustration/anger/distress/embarrassment/concern/withdrawal.

5 Not inappropriate: Upset/frustration/anger/distress/embarrassment/concern/ withdrawal.

47 Wound Care

Identify descriptor that is 'best fit'. The patient/client/student does not have to have each feature mentioned. Use 0.5 to indicate if patient/client/student is slightly better or worse than a descriptor and as appropriate to age.

Impairment

0 Profound. Black/necrotic full thickness wound or large surface area wound, for example burn or large fungating wound with involvement of major blood vessels. Severe continual pain.

1 Deep wound extending to muscle, infected and inflamed or medium surface area wound. Severe pain, some relief with medication.

2 Sloughy wound, subcutaneous damage. Medium exudate, offensive smell. Moderate pain or occasional severe pain, relieved with medication.

3 Granulating clean wound. Epidermal damage, blistered, moist. Pain well controlled.

4 Superficial skin break. Inflamed, reddened area. Occasional discomfort.

5 Skin intact, healthy and pink.

Activity

0 Bed-bound, semi-conscious. Totally dependent.

1 Bed/chair-bound. Requires maximal assistance with all personal activities of daily living

2 Chair-bound, limited mobility. Requires frequent assistance of one person. Can undertake some tasks independently.

3 Mobile with minimum assistance/supervision. Requires some regular nursing intervention.

4 Can live independently. Mainly self-caring with occasional monitoring by other.

5 Totally independent and able to function normally.

Participation

0 Unable to fulfil any social/educational/family role. Not involved in decision making/ no autonomy/no control over environment, no social integration.

1 Low self-confidence/poor self-esteem/limited social integration/socially isolated/ contributes to some basic and limited decisions. Cannot achieve potential in any situation.

2 Some self-confidence/some social integration/makes some decisions and influences control in familiar situations.

3 Some self-confidence; autonomy emerging. Makes decisions and has control of some aspects of life. Able to achieve some limited social integration/educational activities. Diffident over control over life. Needs encouragement to achieve potential.

4 Mostly confident; occasional difficulties integrating or in fulfilling social/role activity. Participates in all appropriate decisions. May have difficulty in achieving potential in some situations occasionally.

5 Achieving potential. Autonomous and unrestricted. Able to fulfil social, educational and family role.

Wellbeing/Distress (client/carer)

0 Severe constant: Upset/frustration/anger/distress/embarrassment/concern/withdrawal. High and constant levels of concern/anger/severe depression/apathy. Unable to express or control emotions appropriately.

1 Frequently severe: Upset/frustration/anger/distress/embarrassment/concern/ withdrawal. Moderate concern, becomes concerned easily, requires constant reassurance/ support, needs clear/tight limits and structure, loses emotional control easily.

2 Moderate consistent: Upset/frustration/anger/distress/embarrassment/concern/ withdrawal. Concern in unfamiliar situation, frequent emotional encouragement and support required.

3 Moderate frequent: Upset/frustration/anger/distress/embarrassment/concern/ withdrawal. Controls emotions with assistance, emotionally dependent on some occasions, vulnerable to change in routine, etc., spontaneously uses methods to assist emotional control.

4 Mild occasional: Upset/frustration/anger/distress/embarrassment/concern/withdrawal. Able to control feelings in most situations, generally well adjusted/stable (most of the time/most situations), occasional emotional support/encouragement needed.

5 Not inappropriate: Upset/frustration/anger/distress/embarrassment/concern/ withdrawal.

New Adapted Scales
Fully Tested

48 Sensory Processing Difficulties

Identify descriptor that is 'best fit'. The patient/client/student does not have to have each feature mentioned. Use 0.5 to indicate if patient/client/student is slightly better or worse than a descriptor and as appropriate to age.

Impairment

0 Profound impairment across multiple sensory systems/specific sensory system(s). Extreme sensitivity to multiple sensory stimuli. Extreme difficulty habituating to sensations or environments. Unable to self-regulate/modulate levels of arousal - extreme fight-and-flight behaviours/high or low arousal. Extremely poor no body awareness/motor planning/ideation. Extreme aggression and/or withdrawal behaviours. Constant sensory seeking, repetitive or ritualistic behaviour observed.

1 Severe impairment across multiple sensory systems/specific sensory system(s). Severe sensitivity to multiple sensory stimuli. Severe difficulty habituating to sensations or environments. Usually unable to self-regulate/modulate levels of arousal - frequent fight-and-flight behaviours/high or low arousal. Severe difficulties with body awareness/motor planning/ideation. Frequent/severe aggression and/or withdrawal behaviours. Frequent sensory seeking, repetitive or ritualistic behaviour.

2 Severe/moderate impairment across multiple sensory systems/specific sensory system(s). Severe/moderate sensitivity to some sensory stimuli. Severe/moderate difficulty habituating to some sensations and/or some environments. Often unable to self-regulate/modulate levels of arousal – commonly displays fight-and-flight behaviours/high or low arousal. Severe/moderate difficulties with body awareness/motor planning/ideation. Often displays aggression and/or withdrawal behaviours. Severe/moderate difficulties focusing/attending to some daily activities. Consistency often varies when performing some daily activities. Some sensory seeking, repetitive or ritualistic behaviour.

3 Moderate impairment across multiple sensory systems/specific sensory system(s). Moderate sensitivity to some sensory stimuli. Moderate difficulty habituating to some sensations and/or environments. Sometimes unable to self-regulate/modulate levels of arousal – sometimes displays fight-and-flight behaviour /high or low arousal. Moderate difficulties with body awareness/motor planning/ideation. Sometimes displays aggression and/or withdrawal behaviours. Moderate difficulties focusing/attending to daily activities. Consistency sometimes varies when performing daily activities. Occasional sensory seeking, repetitive or ritualistic behaviour.

4 Mild impairment across multiple sensory systems/specific sensory system(s). Some mild sensitivity to sensory stimuli. Mild difficulty habituating to a few sensations or environments. Infrequently unable to self-regulate/modulate levels of arousal – rarely displays fight-and-flight behaviours high or low arousal. Occasional mild difficulties with body awareness/motor planning/ideation. Rarely displays aggression and/or withdrawal behaviours. Mild difficulties focusing/attending to daily activities. General consistency when performing daily activities. Rarely demonstrates sensory seeking, repetitive or ritualistic behaviour.

5 No impairment. No observable sensitivity to sensory stimuli. Able to habituate to sensations or environments. Able to self-regulate/modulate levels of arousal – does not display fight-and-flight behaviour /high or low arousal. No difficulties with body awareness/motor planning/ideation (related to sensory difficulties). Does not display aggression and/or withdrawal behaviours (related to sensory difficulties). No difficulties focusing/attending to daily activities. No sensory seeking, repetitive or ritualistic behaviour.

Activity

0 Dependent for all functional tasks. Fully dependent on carers to engage in all activities of daily living. Very poor planning and organization skills. Fully reliant upon care-givers for managing personal safety. Unable to self-initiate or plan tasks effectively. Unable to cope with transitions or change in routine. Difficulty learning new skills. Extreme difficulties focusing/attending to daily activities. Extreme variation in consistency when performing daily activities. Acts on own terms/agenda. No reciprocal play/social skills.

1 Dependent for most tasks but some cooperation. Fully dependent on carers to engage in most activities of daily living but can cooperate with some routines/follow some directions. Poor planning and organization skills. Mostly reliant upon care-givers for managing personal safety. Unable to self-initiate or plan tasks effectively without constant support. Unable to cope with transitions or change in routine. Difficulty learning new skills without repetition/support from a care-giver. Mostly acts on own terms/agenda. No reciprocal play/social skills. Severe/frequent difficulties focusing/attending to daily activities. Frequent variation in consistency when performing daily activities.

2 Needs verbal/physical prompts and support/encouragement to initiate/undertake most tasks. Mainly dependent on carers to engage in activities of daily living but can cooperate with routines/directions. Limited planning and organization skills. Some reliance upon care-givers for managing personal safety. Limited ability to self-initiate or plan tasks effectively without support. Limited ability to cope with transitions or change in routine. Some difficulty learning new skills. Frequently acts on own terms/agenda. Severely limited and rigid in reciprocal play/social skills.

3 Initiates appropriately but needs some support and encouragement to undertake less usual activities. Some dependence on carers to engage in activities of daily living but cooperate with most routines/directions. Some planning and organization skills. Occasional reliance upon care-givers for managing personal safety. Some ability to self-initiate or plan tasks effectively without support. Has ability to cope with transitions or change in routine with support. Occasional difficulty learning new skills. Sometimes acts on own terms/agenda. Lacks flexibility in reciprocal play/social skills in some settings.

4 Able to manage all or nearly all activities of daily living. Mostly independent with activities of daily living and accesses most routines/can follow directions. Generally good planning and organization skills. Can usually manage own personal safety. Can usually self-initiate or plan tasks effectively without support. Can generally cope with transitions or change in routine. Can usually learn new skills without difficulty. Some flexibility with routine and reciprocal play/social skills.

5 Functions normally in all situations. Fully independent with activities of daily living and accesses all routines/can follow directions. Good planning and organization skills. Can manage own personal safety. Can self-initiate or plan tasks effectively without support. Can cope with transitions or change in routine. Can usually learn new skills without difficulty. Able to be flexible with routine/demonstrates consistent reciprocal play/social skills.

Participation

0 No autonomy, isolated, no social/family life. Very limited or non-existent social integration/socially isolated. Unable to participate in family activities or community activities, e.g., shopping or attending an outside event. Unable to make meaningful friendships/relationships with others. Lack of empathy and lack of interest in other people forming relationships with others. Unable to access school-based/employment/recreational and educational activities.

1 Very limited choices, contact mainly with professionals, no social or family role, little control over life. Very limited social integration/socially isolated. Very limited ability to participate in family activities or community activities, e.g., shopping or attending an outside event. Very limited ability to make meaningful friendships/relationships with others. Very limited empathy and lack of interest in other people/forming relationships with others. Very limited ability to access school-based employment/recreational and educational activities.

2 Some integration, value and autonomy. Some limited social integration but mostly socially isolated. Some ability to participate in specific familiar family activities or community activities, e.g., shopping or attending an outside event. Limited ability to make meaningful friendships/relationships with others. Limited empathy and lack of interest in other people/forming relationships with others. Limited ability to access school-based/educational activities.

3 Integrated, valued and autonomous with support. Social integration dependent upon care-giver's support or strategies. Some ability to participate in family activities or community activities, e.g., shopping or attending an outside event with support. Some ability to make meaningful friendships/relationships with others. Can sometimes show empathy and interest in other people/forming relationships with others. Access to school-based/educational activities, with support.

4 Occasionally some restriction in autonomy, integration or role. Social integration with occasional support from care-giver. Ability to participate in most family activities or community activities, e.g., shopping or attending an outside event with support. Usually able to make meaningful friendships/relationships with others. Usually shows empathy and interest in other people/forms relationships with others. Usually accesses school-based/educational activities.

5 Integrated, valued, occupies appropriate role. Socially integrated. Able to participate in family activities or community activities, e.g., shopping or attending an outside event. Able to make meaningful friendships/relationships with others. Shows empathy and interest in other people/forms relationships with others. Accesses school-based/educational activities independently.

Wellbeing/Distress (client/carer)

0 Severe constant: High and constant levels of distress/upset/concern/frustration/anger/embarrassment/withdrawal/severe depression/apathy. Unable to express or control emotions appropriately.

1 Frequently severe: Distress/upset/concern/frustration/anger/embarrassment/withdrawal/severe depression/ apathy. Becomes concerned easily, requires constant reassurance/support, needs clear/tight limits and structure, loses emotional control easily.

2 Moderate frequent: Distress/upset/concern/frustration/anger/withdrawal/severe depression/apathy in unfamiliar situations. Frequent emotional encouragement and support required.

3 Moderate occasional: Distress/upset/concern/frustration/anger/withdrawal/severe depression/apathy. Controls emotions with assistance, emotionally dependent on some occasions, vulnerable to change in routine, etc., spontaneously uses methods to assist emotional control.

4 Mild occasional: Distress/upset/concern/frustration/anger/withdrawal/severe depression/apathy. Able to control feelings in most situations, generally well adjusted/stable (most of the time/most situations), occasional emotional support/encouragement needed.

5 Not inappropriate: Distress/upset/concern/frustration/anger/withdrawal/severe depression/apathy. Well adjusted, stable and able to cope emotionally with most situations, good insight, accepts and understands own limitations.

Acknowledgement: Jamie Liddell in collaboration with Pam Enderby.

49 Chronic Fatigue Syndrome/ME

Identify descriptor that is 'best fit'. The patient/client/student does not have to have each feature mentioned. Use 0.5 to indicate if patient/client/student is slightly better or worse than a descriptor and as appropriate to age.

Impairment

0 Most severe: Persistent severe fatigue, malaise, pain and other symptoms to the extent that the patient requires assistance with all self-care tasks, difficulty mobilizing within the bed to turn over or sit up, and may require assistance with feeding. Difficulty tolerating environmental stimuli such as light, noise, touch, requires masks/ear plugs, etc., or difficulty accepting personal care. Has difficulty with sustaining any minimum communication or cognitive tasks. Concerns about joint mobility and skin integrity due to restricted movement.

1 Severe fatigue, malaise, pain and other symptoms to the extent that the patient is unable to mobilize or carry out any daily task for themselves and is bed-bound the majority of the time. Frequent difficulty tolerating environmental stimuli such as light or noise, requiring significant modification to the environment. Significant cognitive impairment affecting speech and any mental tasks.

2 Severe to moderate fatigue, malaise, pain, sleep impairment and other symptoms to the extent that the patient has reduced mobility which impacts on their ability to leave their home. Frequently requiring assistance, encouragement and reminders related to activities of daily living, including cognitive tasks.

3 Moderate, frequent and fluctuating fatigue, malaise, pain, sleep impairment and other symptoms which worsen after usual daily tasks. Symptoms limit ability to leave the home on occasions. Significant difficulty with memory, word finding and sustaining attention frequently.

4 Mild fatigue, occasional episodes periods of malaise, pain, sleep impairment and other symptoms. Experiences post-exertional malaise when trying to sustain tasks over and above usual daily tasks. Rarely has difficulty with mobility and self-care. Occasionally reports difficulty sustaining cognitive tasks such as word finding, attention and short-term memory when symptoms worsen.

5 No impairment: Able to undertake age-appropriate personal, occupational and social activity required without being limited by post-exertional malaise.

Activity

NB: Level of activity that is sustainable from day to day.

0 Minimal active movement, totally dependent on assistance for all personal care tasks. Confined to bed and unable to sit up/turn over independently. Interaction with the environment, communication tools and others is severely limited.

1 Stays in bed majority of the time but assists or cooperates with caregiver on personal care tasks. Limited purposeful activity and is able to sit up for short periods/roll and turn. Needs assistance with most activities of daily living and transfers. Some awareness and ability to interact and communicate with others.

2 Mobilizes within a familiar indoor environment with support/supervision. Able to initiate some aspects of activities of daily living including self-care tasks. Has some self-management skills and is able to complete some valued activities such as listening to music, reading, electronic communication, cards, etc. May require support with cognitive tasks.

3 Independent in mobility with limitations. Can undertake most activities of daily living independently but requires regular rest periods. Able to plan and carry out a range of day-to-day tasks. Able to complete more complex or demanding tasks with assistance and verbal prompting for shorter periods than usual. Tolerates interaction with others for a limited period.

4 Independently mobile in familiar environments. Independent in all activities of daily living. Needs occasional assistance or extra time to complete demanding physical or complex cognitive tasks. Occasionally requires rest after activity more than is usual for someone without the condition. Adapts activity in response to fluctuations in symptoms and uses self-management techniques.

5 Independent and able to function.

Participation

0 Unable to fulfil any social/educational/work and family roles. No autonomy/isolated with no control over environment.

1 Limited social integration, contact mainly with care-givers, minimal social or family role.

2 Some social integration and occasional decision making limited to familiar situations.

3 Demonstrates autonomy but requires support and assistance to achieve potential. Has control over some aspects of life. Has beliefs in being able to influence environment. Able to fulfil social/educational/work and family roles in a limited capacity.

4 Occasional difficulties integrating or fulfilling social/educational/work and family roles. May have difficulty in achieving potential in certain situations. Able to participate in decision making as required.

5 Achieving potential, fully integrated and autonomous. Able to fulfil social/educational/ work and family roles as appropriate.

Wellbeing/Distress (client/carer)

0 High and constant levels of distress: Unable to express or manage emotions appropriately.

1 Severe levels of distress: Present all or nearly all of the time. Becomes distressed easily and has great difficulty managing emotional reactions, requires constant reassurance/support.

2 Moderate to severe levels of distress: Present most of the time and has difficulty managing emotional reactions. Frequent reassurance/emotional support required.

3 Moderate levels of distress: Occurs regularly but can manage emotional reactions to some degree. Periodically requires reassurance/emotional support.

4 Mild levels of distress: Able to manage feelings in most situations, generally well adjusted/stable but requires occasional emotional support/encouragement.

5 Well adjusted: Able to cope emotionally, good insight, accepts and understands own limitation.

Acknowledgement: Deborah Taylor in collaboration with Pam Enderby.

50 Paediatric Dysphagia

Impairment

0 Profound dysphagia. No detectable swallow on clinical assessment or anatomically unable to achieve oesophageal transit. May have audible pharyngeal pooling of saliva. Consistent, high risk of aspiration or choking.

1 Severe dysphagia. Swallow trigger attempts but ineffective. Limited attempts at rooting, latching or sucking. May show some limited oral control/very late or delayed swallow initiation/very poor pharyngeal clearance/severe laryngeal incompetence/ severe oesophageal dysmotility. Swallow is ineffective for any texture of food or drink. High risk of aspiration or choking.

2 Moderate dysphagia. May show normal non-nutritive sucking, with inadequate/ dysfunctional suck:swallow:breathe synchrony. May show limited oral control/ late or delayed swallow initiation/poor pharyngeal clearance/moderate laryngeal incompetence/oesophageal dysmotility. Oropharyngeal skills are ineffective for some textures. Moderate risk of aspiration or choking.

3 Occasional moderate dysphagia. Secondary to temporary health issues affecting endurance/fatigue/appetite/motivation/experience. May show physiological stress cues. Inconsistent risk of aspiration or choking (can also be used for mild-moderate dysphagia).

4 Mild dysphagia. May show immature suck:swallow:breathe synchrony for gestational age. May show reduced oral control/late or delayed swallow initiation/reduced pharyngeal clearance/mild laryngeal incompetence. Oropharyngeal skills are ineffective or inconsistent for one texture. Occasional risk of aspiration or choking.

5 No difficulty.

Activity

0 Non-oral feeding to meet all hydration and nutritional needs. No oral intake.

1 Non-oral feeding to meet all hydration and nutritional needs. Minimal oral intake, e.g., dummy dips/tastes purée, 5mls or less per feed.

2 Dependent upon non-oral feeding, with consistent intake of food and/or fluid greater than 5mls.

3 Total/mostly oral intake requiring special conditions, e.g., limited volume/frequency/time allowed for oral feed. May need thickened feed, puréed diet where not age appropriate. May need specialist equipment.

4 Total/mostly oral intake requiring minimal support, e.g., using top-ups to support volume required, slow flow teat, side-lying/pacing or avoidance of challenging textures, supportive seating.

5 Age appropriate, fully oral intake.

Participation (if applicable)

Compare with a typically-developing child of similar age, gender and culture. Not applicable for infant under 12 months. Note as 'not assessed'.

0 Unable to participate in family/social/school life. No autonomy/independence or integration in any setting.

1 Very limited participation or ability to make choices in family/social/school life. Very occasionally has some autonomy/integration/independence in one setting.

2 Limited participation in family/social/school life. Limited independence/autonomy and integration in some settings.

3 Integrated, autonomous and independent in a limited number of family/social/school life settings.

4 Occasionally some restriction in participation in family/social/school life and for independence/autonomy and integration.

5 Integrated, valued and autonomous in family/social/school life.

Wellbeing/Distress (rate for parent/carer and, if appropriate, also for the child)

0 Severe, constant: Consistently high levels of distress/anxiety/frustration/confusion.

1 Frequently severe: Frequent, high levels of distress/anxiety/frustration/confusion.

2 Moderate, consistent: Consistent, moderate distress/anxiety/frustration/confusion.

3 Moderate, frequent: Frequent, moderate distress/frustration/anxiety/confusion.

4 Mild, occasional: Occasional, mild distress/frustration/anxiety/confusion.

5 Not distressed.

Acknowledgement: Developed by Bev Curtis. Cardiff and Vale University Health Board in collaboration with Pam Enderby.

Scales in Development

51 Selective Mutism

Scale in development
Identify descriptor that is 'best fit'. The patient/client/student does not have to have each feature mentioned. Use 0.5 to indicate if patient/client/student is slightly better or worse than a descriptor. Consider as appropriate for age, gender and culture.

Impairment

0 Profound selective mutism. Does not speak to anyone, including close family and friends. Characterized by gradual cessation of verbal communication across all settings. Secondary anxiety is displayed as depression, self-harming, social anxiety disorder, social withdrawal, school refusal, aggression or indifference.

1 Severe selective mutism. Does not speak in most social situations, and this pattern is consistent. Speaks to a small number of people associated with a single setting (e.g., home, school). Secondary anxiety is displayed as depression, self-harming, social anxiety disorder, social withdrawal, school refusal, aggression or indifference.

2 Severe/moderate selective mutism. Does not speak in most social situations, and this pattern is consistent. Speaks to a restricted range of people associated with a small number of settings. Displays speech anxiety through muscular tension, low volume, altered voice quality and/or speech avoidance. Secondary anxiety may be displayed as depression, self-harming, social anxiety disorder, social withdrawal, school refusal, aggression or indifference.

3 Moderate selective mutism. Does not speak in some social situations, and this pattern of avoidance is consistent. Failure to speak is linked to one or two settings and the people associated with those settings. Displays speech anxiety in these settings through muscular tension, low volume, altered voice quality and/or speech avoidance. Secondary anxiety may be displayed as separation anxiety, social avoidance, school refusal, hostility or passivity.

4 Mild selective mutism. Speaks in most social situations and settings and this pattern is consistent. Failure to speak is limited to a small number of people and situations involving people in those settings. Usually speaks on a reciprocal basis in other situations. Speech anxiety is usually managed through avoidance.

5 No selective mutism. No evidence of anything but normal anxiety about talking as appropriate to age and experience.

Activity

0 No communication. Does not indicate needs, feelings or opinions through any form of communication.

1 Severely limited communication. Communicates with a restricted range of people on a one-to-one basis. Rarely initiates communication. Rarely communicates needs, feelings or opinions.

2 Limited communication. Communicates with a restricted range of people on a one-to-one and small group basis. Occasionally initiates communication. May respond to questions but does not initiate. Needs support to communicate needs, feelings and opinions in most settings.

3 Functional and effective communication in at least two settings (e.g., family, educational, work or community). May respond to questions but does not initiate communication in other settings/limited communication in other settings. Needs support to communicate needs, feelings and opinions in some settings.

4 Functional communication exhibited in most circumstances and with a broad range of individuals. Contributes verbally to group discussions or conversations. Initiates communication in most settings. Communicates needs, feelings and opinions most of the time. Occasionally exhibits some reticence and requires support to engage. Anticipates a few difficult situations and employs coping/self-help strategies.

5 Communicates verbally and functions appropriately for age in all situations.

Participation

0 No social integration. Not involved in decision making, no autonomy, no control over environment. Unable to reach potential in any situation.

1 Severe difficulties in fulfilling social, educational, work or family roles. Very limited social integration. Very limited involvement in decision making. Very little control over environment. Can only rarely reach potential with support and assistance.

2 Moderately severe difficulties in fulfilling social, educational, work or family roles. Limited social integration. Able to effect some decisions/control in familiar situations. Limited ability to achieve potential and this mostly requires support and assistance.

3 Moderate difficulties in fulfilling social, work, educational or family roles. Able to achieve some social integration. Makes decisions and has control of some aspects of life. Usually reaches potential with or without assistance but frequently needs assistance.

4 Occasional difficulties in fulfilling social/educational/ work/family role. Occasional difficulties with social integration. Participates in all appropriate decisions. May occasionally have difficulty in achieving potential.

5 Able to fulfil social/educational/work/family roles. Autonomous and unrestricted. Achieving potential with no assistance.

Wellbeing/Distress

0 Severe constant: High and constant levels of distress/upset/concern/frustration/anger/ embarrassment/withdrawal/depression or apathy. Unable to express, identify with or control emotions appropriately.

1 Frequently severe: Distress/upset/concern/frustration/anger/embarrassment/ withdrawal/depression/apathy. Can rarely express, identify with or control emotions appropriately.

2 Moderate consistent: Distress/upset/concern/frustration/anger/embarrassment/ withdrawal/depression/apathy. Unable to consistently express or control emotions in most settings. Responds to emotional support.

3 Moderate frequent: Distress/upset/concern/frustration/anger/embarrassment/ withdrawal/depression/apathy. Unable to consistently express or control emotions in some settings. Responds to emotional support.

4 Mild occasional: Distress/upset/concern/frustration/anger/embarrassment/withdrawal/ depression/apathy. Generally well adjusted/stable (most of the time/most situations). Able to express and control emotions appropriately in most situations.

5 Not inappropriate: Distress/upset/concern/frustration/anger/embarrassment/ withdrawal/depression/apathy. Well adjusted, stable and able to cope emotionally with most situations, good insight, accepts and understands own limitations.

Acknowledgement: Developed by Angela Dance, Maggie Johnson, Jeanne Reilly in collaboration with Pam Enderby.

52 Acquired Dyspraxia of Speech

Scale in development
Identify descriptor that is 'best fit'. The patient/client/student does not have to have each feature mentioned. Use 0.5 to indicate if patient/client/student is slightly better or worse than a descriptor. Consider as appropriate for age gender and culture.

Impairment

0 Profound. Unable to imitate any oral movements or sounds. Speech absent or attempts to speak but presents with frequent repetition of unwanted/inappropriate sounds or words. Severe generalized oromotor impairment.

1 Severe. Severely restricted speech system. Can imitate and produce some movements and simple sounds inconsistently and with maximum attention and effort. Consistent groping for articulatory placement and sound production. Frequent repetition of unwanted/inappropriate sounds or words.

2 Severe/moderate impairment. Can imitate and produce automatic words and a restricted range of consonant/vowel combinations. Can imitate some articulatory placements. Accuracy of speech production varies with more incorrect than correct productions. Frequent groping for placement and sound production. Some repetition of unwanted/inappropriate sounds or words.

3 Moderate impairment. Can imitate combined oral motor movements, sounds and words with some inconsistent errors. Can imitate and produce a range of sounds in combination, simple words and phrases with more correct than incorrect productions. Occasional groping for articulatory placement and sound production. Occasional repetition and production of unwanted/inappropriate sounds or words.

4 Mild impairment. Can imitate combined oral movements, compound sound combinations and produce complex sentences with occasional errors. In frequent groping for articulatory placement and sound production. No inappropriate repetition or production of unwanted/inappropriate sounds or words

5 No impairment.

Activity

0 Unable to communicate. No effective communication.

1 Occasionally able to communicate conveying simple and basic needs and wants to familiar persons/trained listeners in familiar contexts with maximum cues and support. May occasionally use limited gestural or other communication method. Constant repetition required. Minimal communication with maximum assistance.

2 Occasional effective communication. Intelligible to familiar listeners with some limitations to functional communication. Able to make basic needs known and contribute to conversation but is dependent on consistent support and familiar listeners in familiar settings. Maintains meaningful interaction related to the here and now with familiar listeners. Repetition required frequently.

3 Consistently able to communicate basic or familiar messages. Some inconsistency in unfamiliar settings or with less usual topics. Is less dependent on cues, gestures and context in order to communicate effectively. Repetition is required occasionally.

4 Mild occasional difficulty with communication experienced in certain (more stressful) situations. Can be understood most the time by any listener even with limitations in the intelligibility. May require consideration by listener, e.g., extra time and attention. Repetition rarely required.

5 Communicates effectively in all situations.

Participation

0 Unable to fulfil any social/educational/family role. Not involved in decision making, no autonomy, no control over environment, no social integration.

1 Low self-confidence, poor self-esteem, limited social integration, socially isolated, contributes to some basic and limited decisions. Cannot achieve potential in any situation.

2 Some self-confidence in familiar situations, some social integration, makes some decisions and influences control in familiar situations.

3 Some self-confidence in broader situations, autonomy emerging. Makes some decisions and influences control in familiar situations. Can fulfil some social, occupational, educational or family role with support from familiar communication partners. Able to make some decisions/control in familiar situations. Needs encouragement to achieve potential.

4 Mostly confident. Occasional difficulties integrating or fulfilling social, occupational and educational activities. Appropriately participates in decision making with little support provided. May have difficulty in achieving potential in unfamiliar situations

5 Achieving potential. Autonomous and unrestricted. Able to fulfil social, educational and family role.

Wellbeing/Distress (client/carer)

0 Severe constant: High and constant levels of distress/upset/concern/frustration/ anger/embarrassment/withdrawal/severe depression/apathy. Unable to express or control emotions appropriately.

1 Frequently severe: Moderate distress/upset/concern/frustration/anger/embarrassment/ withdrawal/severe depression/apathy. Becomes concerned easily, requires constant reassurance/support, needs clear/tight limits and structure, loses emotional control easily.

2 Moderate consistent: Distress/upset/concern/frustration/anger/distress/embarrassment/ withdrawal/severe depression/apathy in unfamiliar situations. Frequent emotional encouragement and support required.

3 Moderate frequent: Distress/upset/concern/frustration/anger/embarrassment/ withdrawal/severe depression/apathy. Controls emotions with assistance, emotionally dependent on some occasions, vulnerable to change in routine, etc., spontaneously uses methods to assist emotional control.

4 Mild occasional: Distress/upset/concern/frustration/anger/embarrassment/withdrawal/ severe depression/apathy. Able to control feelings in most situations, generally well adjusted/stable (most of the time/most situations), occasional emotional support/ encouragement needed.

5 Not inappropriate: Distress/upset/concern/frustration/anger/distress/embarrassment/ withdrawal/severe depression/apathy. Well adjusted, stable and able to cope emotionally with most situations, good insight, accepts and understands own limitations.

Acknowledgement: developed by Aisha O'Gilvie and Elise Minsky in collaboration with Pam Enderby and with the assistance of others.

53 Parent-Infant Responsiveness

Identify descriptor that is 'best fit'. The patient/client/student does not have to have each feature mentioned. Use 0.5 to indicate if patient/client/student is slightly better or worse than a descriptor and as appropriate to age.

Impairment

0 Not aware or identifying readiness cues. Parent does not show any awareness of the baby's engagement and disengagement cues and/or is not able to identify cues in relation to pre-feeding, feeding skills or daily cares.

1 Some awareness and identification of readiness cues. Parent shows some awareness of the baby's engagement and disengagement cues and observed to identify some cues in relation to pre-feeding, feeding skills or daily cares.

2 Limited awareness and identification of readiness cues. Parent shows limited awareness of engagement OR disengagement cues and observed to identify or give example of cues during single care only in relation to pre-feeding, feeding skills or daily cares.

3 Inconsistent awareness and identification of readiness cues. Parent shows inconsistent awareness of engagement OR disengagement cues and observed to identify cues or be able to give clear examples in relation to pre-feeding, feeding skills or daily cares.

4 Consistent awareness and identification of readiness cues. Parent shows consistent awareness of engagement AND disengagement and observed to identify cues or able to give clear examples in relation to most pre-feeding, feeding skills and daily cares.

5 Competent awareness and identification of readiness cues. Parent shows competent awareness of engagement AND disengagement cues and observed to show full autonomy in identifying cues in relation to pre-feeding, feeding skills and daily cares.

Activity

0 No adaptation: Parent shows no adaptation in their interaction with the baby during any pre-feeding, feeding or daily cares when engagement AND disengagement signs observed. Needs experienced supervision.

1 Restricted adaptation: Parent shows adaptation in one interaction with the baby during pre-feeding, feeding or daily care when engagement OR disengagement cues are observed. Needs experienced supervision.

2 Limited adaptation: Parent shows adaptation in more than one interaction with the baby during pre-feeding, feeding or daily care when engagement OR disengagement cues are observed. Needs experienced supervision.

3 Inconsistent supported adaptation: Parent shows adaptation in their interaction with the baby during more than one pre-feeding, feeding or daily care when engagement OR disengagement cues are observed. Requires experienced supervision to adapt interactions appropriately.

4 Consistent supported adaptation: Parent shows spontaneous adaptation in multiple interactions with the baby during familiar pre-feeding, feeding and daily cares when engagement AND disengagement cues are observed. Needs occasional experienced supervision to adapt interactions appropriately.

5 Competent autonomous adaptation: Parent shows spontaneous autonomous adaptation of all interactions with the baby during pre-feeding, feeding and daily cares when engagement AND disengagement signs are observed. No further support indicated.

Participation

0 Unable to fulfil any social/educational/family role. Not involved in decision-making/ no autonomy, no control over environment, no integration in mealtimes.

1 Low self-confidence, poor self-esteem, limited social integration in mealtimes, socially isolated, contributes to some basic and limited decisions. Cannot achieve potential in any situation.

2 Some self-confidence, some social integration during mealtimes, makes some decisions & influences control in familiar situations.

3 Some self-confidence, autonomy emerging. Makes decisions and has control of some aspects of life. Able to achieve some limited social integration during mealtimes. Diffident over control over life. Needs encouragement to achieve potential.

4 Mostly confident, occasional difficulties integrating or in fulfilling social/role activity. Participating in all appropriate decisions. May have difficulty in achieving potential in some situations occasionally.

5 Achieving potential. Autonomous and unrestricted. Able to fulfil social, educational and family role.

Wellbeing/Distress (rate for parent/carer and, if appropriate, also for the infant)

0 Severe constant: High and constant levels of distress/upset/concern/frustration/ anger/embarrassment/withdrawal/severe depression/apathy. Unable to express or control emotions appropriately.

1 Frequently severe: Moderate distress/upset/concern/frustration/anger/embarrassment/withdrawal/severe depression/apathy. Becomes concerned easily, requires constant reassurance/support, needs clear/tight limits and structure, loses emotional control easily.

2 Moderate consistent: Distress/upset/concern/frustration/anger/embarrassment/withdrawal/severe depression/apathy in unfamiliar situations, frequent emotional encouragement and support required.

3 Moderate frequent: Distress/upset/concern/frustration/anger/embarrassment/withdrawal/severe depression/apathy. Controls emotions with assistance, emotionally dependent on some occasions, vulnerable to change in routine, etc., spontaneously uses methods to assist emotional control.

4 Mild occasional: Distress/upset/concern/frustration/anger/embarrassment/withdrawal/severe depression/apathy. Able to control feelings in most situations, generally well-adjusted/stable (most of the time/most situations), occasional emotional support/encouragement needed.

5 Not inappropriate: Distress/upset/concern/frustration/anger/embarrassment/withdrawal/severe depression/apathy. Well adjusted, stable and able to cope emotionally

Acknowledgement: M Peck and A Connolly (2019) Royal London Children's Hospital

54 Oral Hygiene

Identify descriptor that is 'best fit'. The patient/client/student does not have to have each feature mentioned. Use 0.5 to indicate if patient/client/student is slightly better or worse than a descriptor and as appropriate to age.

Impairment

0 Profoundly unhealthy oral mucosa, with evidence of widespread wet or dried, thick mucous and/or blood plaques or food debris. Open ulcerations/bleeding, blistered tongue. Clinical signs of infection.

1 Severely unhealthy oral mucosa, with evidence of persistent generalized plaques, food debris, thick coating of mucous or blood on oral structures, recurrent ulcers/blisters. High and constant risk of infection.

2 Severe/moderately unhealthy status of oral mucosa, has specific severe difficulty in maintaining more than one element of healthy oral mucosa, e.g., widespread oral thrush, cracked lips, inflammation, food debris. At regular risk of infection.

3 Moderately unhealthy status of oral mucosa requires regular oral hygiene programme. May have specific more severe difficulty in maintaining one element of healthy oral mucosa, e.g., food debris, coated tongue, dry lips, localized oral thrush or debris to one structure.

4 Mild status of oral mucosa, healthy oral mucosa but may require increased frequency of mouth care.

5 Healthy oral mucosa, pink, perfuse, moist and clean.

Activity

0 Medicated specialist high frequency oral hygiene programme to meet oral hygiene needs. Two-hourly mouth care programme. Using multiple medicated and non-medicated specialist protocols, e.g., medicated mouthwash, topical medication, oral thrush medication, oral saliva replacement gel or spray *and* suction toothbrush and/or yankeur suction.

1 Non-medicated specialist high frequency oral hygiene programme to meet oral hygiene needs. Two-hourly mouth care programme using multiple non-medicated specialist protocols, e.g., suction toothbrush and/or yankeur suction, non-foaming toothpaste.

2 Specialist moderate frequency oral hygiene programme to meet oral hygiene needs. Four-to-six hourly mouth care programme using more than one specialist protocol, e.g. ,suction toothbrush and/or yankeur suction, non-foaming toothpaste.

3 Adapted oral hygiene programme to meet oral hygiene needs. Two-to-three times daily mouth care programme. Requires one specialist protocol, e.g., non-foaming toothpaste.

4 Regular oral hygiene programme to meet oral hygiene needs, e.g., increased frequency.

5 Universal oral hygiene plan only, e.g., 2 times daily tooth brushing with fluoride toothpaste.

Participation

0 Unable to fulfil any social/ educational/ family role. Not involved in decision making/ no autonomy, no control over environment, no social integration.

1 Low self-confidence, poor self-esteem, limited social integration, socially isolated, contributes to some basic and limited decisions. Cannot achieve potential in any situation.

2 Some self-confidence, some social integration, makes some decisions and influences control in familiar situations.

3 Some self-confidence, autonomy emerging. Makes decisions and has control of some aspects of life. Able to achieve some limited social integration/educational activities. Diffident over control over life. Needs encouragement to achieve potential.

4 Mostly confident, occasional difficulties integrating or in fulfilling social/role activity. Participates in all appropriate decisions. May have difficulty in achieving potential in some situations occasionally.

5 Achieving potential. Autonomous and unrestricted. Able to fulfil social, educational and family role.

Wellbeing/Distress

0 Severe constant: High and constant levels of distress/upset/concern/frustration/ anger/embarrassment/withdrawal/severe depression/apathy. Unable to express or control emotions appropriately.

1 Frequently severe: Moderate distress/upset/concern/frustration/anger/embarrassment/ withdrawal/severe depression/apathy. Becomes concerned easily, requires constant reassurance/support, needs clear/tight limits and structure, loses emotional control easily.

2 Moderate consistent: Distress/upset/concern/frustration/anger/embarrassment/ withdrawal/severe depression/apathy in unfamiliar situations, frequent emotional encouragement and support required.

3 Moderate frequent: Distress/upset/concern/frustration/anger/embarrassment/ withdrawal/severe depression/apathy. Controls emotions with assistance, emotionally dependent on some occasions, vulnerable to change in routine, etc., spontaneously uses methods to assist emotional control.

4 Mild occasional: Distress/upset/concern/frustration/anger/embarrassment/withdrawal/ severe depression/apathy. Able to control feelings in most situations, generally well adjusted/stable (most of the time/most situations), occasional emotional support/ encouragement needed.

5 Not inappropriate: Distress/upset/concern/frustration/anger/embarrassment/ withdrawal/severe depression/apathy. Well adjusted, stable and able to cope emotionally

Written by Paediatric SLTs M. Peck, K. Jones, and E. O'Dwyer in consultation with Paediatric Dental Team, Royal London Children's Hospital, 2019.

55 Oral Aversion

Identify descriptor that is 'best fit'. The patient/client/student does not have to have each feature mentioned. Use 0.5 to indicate if patient/client/student is slightly better or worse than a descriptor and as appropriate to age.

Impairment

0 Profound oral aversion. Immediate signs of stress, retching, vomiting, +/- physiological instability upon sight or smell of food , dummy or eating and drinking utensils.

1 Severe oral aversion. Accepts dry dummy/spoon in own mouth. May suck on own fingers/hand with no evidence of aversion. Gags/retches when spoon moves further into mouth.

2 Severe/moderate oral aversion. Accepts dry or coated dummy/spoon in own mouth. May suck on own fingers/hand with no evidence of aversion. Gags, retches, increased distress when fluids or solids are introduced.

3 Moderate oral aversion. Accepts small weaning spoons or small amounts of puree on fingers or hands. May take dry spoon to mouth. Signs of stress observed when adult approaches with spoon, e.g., turning away, grimacing, distress. Requires some supplementation with diet and monitoring of weight.

4 Mild oral aversion. Able to feed self or be fed by an adult without any signs of stress. Some selectivity with textures (solids) and +/- reduced quantity. May self-limit with fluids. No concerns regarding nutritional intake or weight gain.

5 No evidence of oral aversion. Eats and drinks a wide range of foods from all nutritional groups. Any selectivity is within normal limits for age. No concerns regarding nutritional intake or weight gain.

Activity

0 Non-oral feeding to meet all hydration and nutritional needs. Not able to participate in oral trials.

1 Non-oral feeding to meet all hydration and nutritional needs. Variable response to oral trials. Needs experienced mealtime partner.

2 Non-oral feeding/supplements needed to meet hydration and nutritional needs. Consistently able to participate in oral trials. Needs experienced mealtime partner.

3 Consistently able to take small quantities of solids and fluids. Needs some adult support. May require feeding supplements for nutrition and/or weight. May eat extremely slowly.

4 Although food selectivity is observed, it is good enough to meet nutritional requirements. Minimal supportive strategies needed. May take a little extra time and avoid certain foods, drinks, or eating situations.

5 Functionally eating and drinking a range of textures from all three food groups.

Participation

0 Unable to fulfil any social/ educational/ family role. Not involved in decision making/ no autonomy, no control over environment, no integration in mealtimes.

1 Low self-confidence, poor self-esteem, limited social integration in mealtimes, socially isolated, contributes to some basic and limited decisions. Cannot achieve potential in any situation.

2 Some self-confidence, some social integration during mealtimes, makes some decisions and influences control in familiar situations.

3 Some self-confidence, autonomy emerging. Makes decisions and has control of some aspects of life. Able to achieve some limited social integration during mealtimes. Diffident over control over life. Needs encouragement to achieve potential.

4 Mostly confident, occasional difficulties integrating or in fulfilling social/role activity. Participates in all appropriate decisions. May have difficulty in achieving potential in some situations occasionally.

5 Achieving potential. Autonomous and unrestricted. Able to fulfil social, educational and family role.

Wellbeing/Distress

0 Severe constant: High and constant levels of distress/upset/concern/frustration/ anger/embarrassment/withdrawal/severe depression/apathy. Unable to express or control emotions appropriately.

1 Frequently severe: Moderate distress/upset/concern/frustration/anger/embarrassment/ withdrawal/severe depression/apathy. Becomes concerned easily, requires constant reassurance/support, needs clear/tight limits and structure, loses emotional control easily.

2 Moderate consistent: Distress/upset/concern/frustration/anger/embarrassment/ withdrawal/severe depression/apathy in unfamiliar situations, frequent emotional encouragement and support required.

3 Moderate frequent: Distress/upset/concern/frustration/anger/embarrassment/ withdrawal/severe depression/apathy. Controls emotions with assistance, emotionally dependent on some occasions, vulnerable to change in routine, etc., spontaneously uses methods to assist emotional control.

4 Mild occasional: Distress/upset/concern/frustration/anger/embarrassment/withdrawal/ severe depression/apathy. Able to control feelings in most situations, generally well adjusted/stable (most of the time/most situations), occasional emotional support/ encouragement needed.

5 Not inappropriate: Distress/upset/concern/frustration/anger/embarrassment/ withdrawal/severe depression/apathy. Well adjusted, stable and able to cope emotionally.

Acknowledgement: Developed by M Peck and A Connolly (2019), Royal London Children's Hospital, collaborating with Pam Enderby.

56 Orthopaedic: Hip and Knee Surgery

Scale in development
Identify descriptor that is 'best fit'. The patient/client/student does not have to have each feature mentioned. Use 0.5 to indicate if patient/client/student is slightly better or worse than a descriptor. Consider as appropriate for age gender and culture.

Impairment

0 Profound. Severe and constant pain, numbness/parathesia (including foot drop), non-weight bearing, severe leg length discrepancy unable to be corrected.

1 Severe impairment. Constant pain not controlled by pain relief, severe consistent neurological signs, non-weight bearing, severe leg length discrepancy requiring onward referral.

2 Moderate impairment. Inhibiting pain, moderate consistent neurological signs, brief touch weight bearing, moderate leg length discrepancy requiring onward referral.

3 Mild impairment. Intermittent pain, mild consistent neurological signs, touch weight bearing, minimal leg length discrepancy requiring onward referral.

4 Slight impairment: Occasional discomfort, mild intermittent neurological signs, partial weight bearing, minimal leg length discrepancy does not require onward referral.

5 No impairment. No pain, no neurological signs, full weight bearing, no leg length discrepancy.

Activity

0 Immobile. Totally dependent in all/any environments. Unable to participate in tasks. Unable to mobilize. Fully dependent on others for personal care.

1 Severe impairment. Requires maximum assistance for all transfers using equipment and assistance of 2, transfers only. Able to participate minimally in personal care.

2 Moderate impairment. Transfers with equipment and assistance of 1, mobile short distance with walking equipment. Needs assistance for personal care.

3 Mild impairment. Transfers with equipment and supervision only. Mobile with walking equipment around home needing rest periods. Supervision and some assistance for personal care.

4 Slight impairment. Transfers with equipment independently. Mobilizes with walking equipment around home comfortably. Occasional assistance for personal care.

5 Independent. Able to transfer independently with no equipment. Mobilizes unaided indoors, able to mobilize outdoors. Independent in all activities.

Participation

0 No participation. Unable to make decisions, unable/unwilling to participate in any activities, socially isolated.

1 Limited participation. Very limited choices made, little control over life, little to no family or social contact, not achieving potential in any situation.

2 Some participation. Able to make some choices, some influence on daily life in familiar settings, some family/social contact, shows interest in participation in previous activities.

3 Some confidence: Makes choices and has some control over daily life, limited social interaction, needs encouragement and support to participate in any activity.

4 Mostly confident: Able to make choices and decisions in differing situations, increased social interaction within the home, social interaction outside of the home – needs occasional assistance and encouragement.

5 Full participation. Confidently makes decisions in daily life, resumes previous activity levels.

Wellbeing/Distress (client/carer)

0 Severe constant: High and constant levels of distress/upset/concern/frustration/anger/embarrassment/withdrawal/severe depression/apathy. Unable to express or control emotions appropriately.

1 Frequently severe: Moderate distress/upset/concern/frustration/anger/embarrassment/withdrawal/severe depression/apathy. Becomes concerned easily, requires constant reassurance/support, needs clear/tight limits and structure, loses emotional control easily.

2 Moderate consistent: Distress/upset/concern/frustration/anger/embarrassment/withdrawal/severe depression/apathy in unfamiliar situations. Frequent emotional encouragement and support required.

3 Moderate frequent: Distress/upset/concern/frustration/anger/embarrassment/withdrawal/severe depression/apathy. Controls emotions with assistance, emotionally dependent on some occasions, vulnerable to change in routine, etc., spontaneously uses methods to assist emotional control.

4 Mild occasional: Distress/upset/concern/frustration/anger/embarrassment/withdrawal/severe depression/apathy. Able to control feelings in most situations, generally well adjusted/stable (most of the time/most situations), occasional emotional support/encouragement needed.

5 Not inappropriate: Distress/upset/concern/frustration/anger/embarrassment/withdrawal/severe depression/apathy. Well adjusted, stable and able to cope emotionally with most situations, good insight, accepts and understands own limitations

Acknowledgement: Developed by Naomi Moore in collaboration with Pam Enderby.

57 Acquired Motor Dyspraxia

Scale in development
Identify descriptor that is 'best fit'. The patient/client/student does not have to have each feature mentioned. Use 0.5 to indicate if patient/client/student is slightly better or worse than a descriptor. Consider as appropriate for age gender and culture.

Impairment

0 Profound problems evident in all areas of sensory-motor skills, including vestibular, sensory processing and modulation, movement and task planning and organization, balance and coordination. Severe perceptual and ideational difficulties. Severe generalized/motor impairment. Very limited attention to tasks.

1 Severe problems usually involving all areas as indicated above, or may involve severe problems in two or more areas or one profound overriding problem, for example severe sensory defensiveness or motor impairment.

2 Severe/moderate impairment in some areas, may involve one severe overriding area, for example gross or fine motor skills, perception, coordination, handwriting or movement planning.

3 Moderate impairment in some areas and/or specific moderate problems in one area, such as motor skills, organization, concentration, writing or perception.

4 Mild impairment in one or more areas involving fine or gross motor skills, perception, coordination, attention, praxis.

5 No impairment, functions at pre-morbid level.

Activity

0 Unable to function independently in any way. Unable to perform any activity without skilled and continual assistance, specialized equipment, supervision or simplification.

1 Occasionally able to perform some simple/automatic activities independently, or to perform some small parts of some tasks alone. Minimal function with maximum assistance.

2 Able to perform basic simple tasks or parts of more complex tasks. Works better with a familiar carer, but lacks confidence or ability in unfamiliar situations. Difficulty learning new skills or transferring them to different situations. Verbal prompts help.

3 Consistently able to perform simple tasks or parts of more complex tasks without help. Can occasionally attempt new tasks building on existing skills. Needs help for some activities, or extra time, or tasks to be broken down or simplified. Verbal prompting may be needed.

4 Occasional difficulties experienced in certain situations or with certain activities. May require extra time to complete tasks. Occasional verbal prompts may be helpful.

5 Functions well in all situations and is fully independent.

Participation

0 Unable to fulfil any social/educational/family role. Not involved in decision making, no autonomy, no control over environment, no social integration.

1 Low self-confidence, poor self-esteem, limited social integration, socially isolated, contributes to some basic and limited decisions. Cannot achieve potential in any situation.

2 Some self-confidence, some social integration, makes some decisions and influences control in familiar situations.

3 Some self-confidence, autonomy emerging. Makes decisions and has control of some aspects of life. Able to achieve some limited social integration/educational activities. Diffident over control over life. Needs encouragement to achieve potential.

4 Mostly confident, occasional difficulties integrating or in fulfilling social/role activity. Participates in all appropriate decisions. May have difficulty in achieving potential in some situations occasionally.

5 Achieving potential. Autonomous and unrestricted. Able to fulfil social, educational and family role.

Wellbeing/Distress (client/carer)

0 Severe constant: High and constant levels of distress/upset/concern/frustration/ anger/embarrassment/withdrawal/severe depression/apathy. Unable to express or control emotions appropriately.

1 Frequently severe: Moderate distress/upset/concern/frustration/anger/embarrassment/ withdrawal/severe depression/apathy. Becomes concerned easily, requires constant reassurance/support, needs clear/tight limits and structure, loses emotional control easily.

2 Moderate consistent: Distress/upset/concern/frustration/anger/embarrassment/ withdrawal/severe depression/apathy in unfamiliar situations. Frequent emotional encouragement and support required.

3 Moderate frequent: Distress/upset/concern/frustration/anger/embarrassment/ withdrawal/severe depression/apathy. Controls emotions with assistance, emotionally dependent on some occasions, vulnerable to change in routine, etc., spontaneously uses methods to assist emotional control.

4 Mild occasional: Distress/upset/concern/frustration/anger/embarrassment/withdrawal/ severe depression/apathy. Able to control feelings in most situations, generally well adjusted/stable (most of the time/most situations), occasional emotional support/ encouragement needed.

5 Not inappropriate: Distress/upset/concern/frustration/anger/embarrassment/ withdrawal/severe depression/apathy. Well adjusted, stable and able to cope emotionally with most situations, good insight, accepts and understands own limitations.

Acknowledgement: Developed by Jenny Evans in collaboration with Pam Enderby.

58 Transgender: Communication

Scale in development
Identify descriptor that is 'best fit'. The patient/client/student does not have to have each feature mentioned. Use 0.5 to indicate if patient/client/student is slightly better or worse than a descriptor. Consider as appropriate for age gender and culture.

Impairment

0 Profound. Presents completely in previous gender with regard to voice, vegetative sounds, verbal mannerisms, body language, physical appearance.

1 Severe. Presents as either previous gender or androgynous with regard to voice, vegetative sounds, verbal mannerisms, body language, physical appearance.

2 Severe-moderate. Presents in new gender in one feature, and androgynous in others with regard to voice, vegetative sounds, verbal mannerisms, body language, physical appearance. May still present as previous gender in one feature.

3 Moderate. Presents in new gender in several features and androgynous in others with regard to voice, vegetative sounds, verbal mannerisms, body language, physical appearance.

4 Mild. Good presentation in all features in virtually all situations with regard to voice, vegetative sounds, verbal mannerisms, body language, physical appearance.

5 Presents fully in new gender with regard to voice, vegetative sounds, verbal mannerisms, body language, physical appearance.

Activity

0 Not able to perform any gender-specific activities in new gender.

1 Able to perform a few gender-specific activities in new gender with difficulty.

2 Able to perform some gender-specific activities in new gender with difficulty.

3 Able to perform some gender-specific activities in new gender with ease.

4 Able to perform most gender-specific activities in new gender with ease.

5 Able to perform all gender-specific activities in new gender with ease.

Participation

0 No autonomy, isolated, no social/family life.

1 Very limited choices, contact mainly with professionals, no social or family role, little control over life.

2 Some integration, value and autonomy in one setting.

3 Integrated, valued and autonomous in limited number of settings.

4 Occasionally some restriction in autonomy, integration or role.

5 Integrated, valued, occupies appropriate role.

Wellbeing/Distress (client/carer)

0 Severe constant: High and constant levels of distress/upset/concern/frustration/anger/embarrassment/withdrawal/severe depression/apathy. Unable to express or control emotions appropriately.

1 Frequently severe: Moderate distress/upset/concern/frustration/anger/embarrassment/withdrawal/severe depression/apathy. Becomes concerned easily, requires constant reassurance/support, needs clear tight limits and structure, loses emotional control easily.

2 Moderate consistent: Distress/upset/concern/frustration/anger/embarrassment/withdrawal/severe depression/apathy in unfamiliar situations. Frequent emotional encouragement and support required.

3 Moderate frequent: Distress/upset/concern/frustration/anger/embarrassment/withdrawal/severe depression/apathy. Controls emotions with assistance, emotionally dependent on some occasions, vulnerable to changes in routine, etc., spontaneously uses methods to assist emotional control.

4 Mild occasional: Distress/upset/concern/frustration/anger/embarrassment/withdrawal/severe depression/apathy. Able to control feelings in most situations, generally well adjusted/stable (most of the time/most situations), occasional emotional support/encouragement needed

5 Not inappropriate: Distress/upset/concern/frustration/anger/embarrassment/withdrawal/severe depression/apathy. Well adjusted, stable and able to cope emotionally with most situations, good insight, accepts and understands own limitations

Acknowledgement: Developed by Jenny Evans, Eimear McCrory, Lyn Johnston in collaboration with Pam Enderby.

59 Trismus

Scale in development
Identify descriptor that is 'best fit'. The patient/client/student does not have to have each feature mentioned. Use 0.5 to indicate if patient/client/student is slightly better or worse than a descriptor. Consider as appropriate for age gender and culture.

Impairment

NB Maximum incisional opening (MIO) is normally measured tooth-to-tooth. For tooth-to-gum add 5mm to scores, for gum-to-gum add 10mm. Where pain scores and jaw opening scores differ, score the most severe.

0 Profound. MIO of 0–9mm. Profound/constant pain.

1 Severe. MIO of 10–15mm. Severe/frequent pain.

2 Severe moderate. MIO of 16–20mm. Strong/frequent discomfort.

3 Moderate. MIO of 21–25mm. Moderate/occasional discomfort.

4 Mild. MIO of 26–34 mm. Mild/infrequent discomfort.

5 Normal. MIO of 35mm or more. No discomfort.

Activity

0 Profound/severe impact on ability to clean teeth, eat, speak, etc.

1 Severe impact, requires, e.g., puréed food, can only clean incisors.

2 Moderate/severe impact, needing to use stretches before attempting eating, can chew some foods.

3 Moderate impact, can use small toothbrush, cuts food up small.

4 Can clean teeth with mild difficulty and chew most foods.

5 Full function. Only needs to carry out stretch regime once a day.

Participation

0 No autonomy, isolated, no social/family life.

1 Very limited choices, contact mainly with professionals, no social or family role, little control over life.

2 Some integration, value and autonomy in one setting.

3 Integrated, valued and autonomous in limited number of settings.

4 Occasionally some restriction in autonomy, integration or role.

5 Integrated, valued, occupies appropriate role.

Wellbeing/Distress (client/carer)

0 Severe constant: High and constant levels of distress/upset/concern/frustration/ anger/embarrassment/withdrawal/severe depression/apathy. Unable to express or control emotions appropriately.

1 Frequently severe: Moderate distress/upset/concern/frustration/anger/embarrassment/ withdrawal/severe depression/apathy. Becomes concerned easily, requires constant reassurance/support, needs clear/tight limits and structure, loses emotional control easily.

2 Moderate consistent: Distress/upset/concern/frustration/anger/embarrassment/ withdrawal/severe depression/apathy in unfamiliar situations, frequent emotional encouragement and support required.

3 Moderate frequent: Distress/upset/concern/frustration/anger/embarrassment/ withdrawal/severe depression/apathy. Controls emotions with assistance, emotionally dependent on some occasions, vulnerable to changes in routine, etc., spontaneously uses methods to assist emotional control.

4 Mild occasional: Distress/upset/concern/frustration/anger/embarrassment/withdrawal/ severe depression/apathy. Able to control feelings in most situations, generally well adjusted/stable (most of the time/most situations), occasional emotional support/ encouragement needed.

5 Not inappropriate: Distress/upset/concern/frustration/anger/embarrassment/ withdrawal/severe depression/apathy. Well adjusted, stable and able to cope emotionally with most situations, good insight, accepts and understands own limitations.

Acknowledgement: Developed by Jenny Evans in collaboration with Pam Enderby.

60 Cognitive Communication Disorder

Scale in development
Identify descriptor that is 'best fit'. The patient/client/student does not have to have each feature mentioned. Use 0.5 to indicate if patient/client/student is slightly better or worse than a descriptor and as appropriate to age.

Impairment

0 Profound. Unresponsive to most stimuli. Does not recognize people, unable to attend or concentrate. Severe disorientation, severely impaired short- and long-term memory. No communicative intent. Severely impaired comprehension and expression. No sense of time or place. Inability to respond to external stimuli.

1 Severe. Some occasional basic communicative intent, e.g., making vocal or nonverbal requests to meet needs or in response. Occasionally able to communicate basic needs. Delayed or inconsistent response to some stimuli. Occasionally responds to some simple commands associated with the present. Obvious disorientation with significantly impaired short-term memory, impaired long-term memory. Occasionally recognizes familiar people or routine tasks in context.

2 Severe/moderate. Occasionally responds appropriately to stimuli, and simple commands, able to understand some simple instructions within context and occasionally expresses appropriately through verbal/nonverbal communication issues to do with the here and now. Moderate to severe inattention. Able to recognize relationships in context more consistently. Use of language may be socially inappropriate with limited understanding of social rules.

3 Moderate. Recognizes familiar people and tasks in most contexts. Orientated to familiar environments with structure. Able to comprehend everyday conversation within context. Recognizes relationships. Able to express immediate needs but may have expressive difficulties. May misunderstand quick or more complex communication. Nonverbal and verbal communication deficits are obvious to a non-skilled observer, e.g., vocal tone, random vocalization, misunderstanding, limited or abnormal facial expression. Frequently repetitive.

4 Mild. Difficulties in communication are subtle. Communication style may be rigid and not necessarily natural/automatic. Orientated in time and place. Has insight into communication disorder and uses strategies to improve communication in familiar environments but may require repetition and more time. Able to understand most complex conversation but requires repetition and further explanation. May have some expressive difficulties, difficulties with comprehending in stressful environments or when fatigued. May have tendency to repeat. Manages a range of surroundings and changes in routines.

5 No disorder. Good age-appropriate comprehension, expression, reading and writing and social responses.

Activity

0 No purposeful communication. Unable to communicate in any way. May be frequently distressed and have totally disruptive and uncooperative behaviour. Inability to recognize and respond appropriately to bodily/biological needs, e.g., thirst/hunger/toileting/pain/temperature, etc. Unable to reliably communicate needs at any time and in any meaningful way.

1 Some slight awareness and recognition of/to communicate. Requires prompting to be involved in even basic communication. Occasionally initiates basic communication. Some minimal attempt to participate in communication. Some nonverbal and verbal attempts may be interpreted by familiar assistants. Occasionally able to make needs understood through verbal/nonverbal communication due to familiarity with situation or an individual.

2 Requires physical and/or verbal prompting and support to plan, initiate, complete or sustain purposeful interaction and communication. Limited spontaneous functional communication but can occasionally make views and basic needs understood. Unable to conduct a flowing conversation. Communicates more consistently with persons who are familiar with their communication style. Frequent repetition required. Some meaningful interaction related to here and now.

3 Initiates communication appropriately. Recognizes and responds appropriately to needs in a familiar environment. Consistently able to make needs known but is inconsistent in less familiar settings. May have significant difficulty with paralinguistic features. May need support to plan/initiate/sustain purposeful communication. Requires assistance for more complex communicative activities.

4 Able to be independent in most communicative activities but need support and encouragement to undertake less familiar or usual tasks. May require occasional prompts/reminders and/or modifications to maintain performance. Able to understand most complex conversation but requires repetition and further explanation. May have difficulty with subtleties of verbal and nonverbal communication and difficulty appreciating humour, sarcasm and irony. Can use strategies. Communicates well most of the time and with a wide range of people.

5 Age-appropriate communication in all situations.

Participation

0 Unable to fulfil any social/educational/family role. Unable to participate in decision making, no autonomy, no control over environment, no social integration.

1 Low self-confidence, poor self-esteem, limited social integration, socially isolated, contributes to some basic and limited decisions. Cannot achieve potential in any situation. Few relationships outside immediate family. Only able to engage in social activities with considerable support from others.

2 Some self-confidence, some social integration, makes some decisions and influences control but only in in familiar situations. May be unable to predict consequences/outcomes of decisions. Able to engage more readily in some limited social integration but social/recreational life is limited. Able to respond to and seek some social integration but requires support to recognize social boundaries.

3 Makes decisions and has control over some aspects of life, autonomy emerging. Understands potential consequences. Able to achieve some limited social integration/recreation/social/educational activities. Insight and concern over social participation. Needs encouragement to achieve potential.

4 Confident and autonomous in most activities. Occasional difficulties integrating or in fulfilling social/role activity. Participates in all appropriate decisions. Occasionally has difficulty in achieving potential in some less familiar situations.

5 Achieving potential. Autonomous and unrestricted. Able to fulfil social, educational and family role.

Wellbeing/Distress (client/carer)

0 Severe constant: High and constant levels of distress/upset/concern/frustration/anger/embarrassment/withdrawal/severe depression/apathy. Unable to express or control emotions appropriately.

1 Frequently severe: Moderate distress/upset/concern/frustration/anger/embarrassment/withdrawal/severe depression/apathy. Becomes concerned easily, requires constant reassurance/support, needs clear/tight limits and structure, loses emotional control easily.

2 Moderate consistent: Distress/upset/concern/frustration/anger/embarrassment/withdrawal/severe depression/apathy in unfamiliar situations. Frequent emotional encouragement and support required.

3 Moderate frequent: Distress/upset/concern/frustration/anger/embarrassment/withdrawal/severe depression/apathy. Controls emotions with assistance, emotionally dependent on some occasions, vulnerable to change in routine, etc., spontaneously uses methods to assist emotional control.

4 Mild occasional: Distress/upset/concern/frustration/anger/embarrassment/withdrawal/severe depression/apathy. Able to control feelings in most situations, generally well adjusted/stable (most of the time/most situations), occasional emotional support/encouragement needed.

5 Not inappropriate: Distress/upset/concern/frustration/anger/embarrassment/withdrawal/severe depression/apathy. Well adjusted, stable and able to cope emotionally with most situations, good insight, accepts and understands own limitations.

Acknowledgement: Pam Enderby with Tery Killick.

61 Velopharyngeal Dysfunction

The individual does not have to have each feature mentioned in the descriptor. It is a best-fit description, i.e. does this description fit the individual better than the other one? Use the 0.5 to indicate if the individual is slightly better or worse than the descriptor. Consider as appropriate for age.

Impairment 1: Velopharyngeal function

0 Profound impairment. Severe hypernasality on vowels with no oral consonants.

1 Severe impairment. Severe hypernasal tone with some attempts at oral consonants. Airflow errors and/or grimace accompanying all high pressure consonants.

2 Moderate impairment. Moderate hypernasality affecting all vowels. Airflow errors affecting more than 3 consonants.

3 Mild impairment. Mild consistent hypernasality and/or airflow errors affecting 1-2 consonants.

4 Borderline. Occasional and inconsistent hypernasality and/or airflow errors.

5 Clear speech. Normal resonance and airflow. Oral tone with good pressure to consonants and no airflow errors.

Impairment 2: Articulation

0 Profound. Totally limited sound system. Uses no recognizable consonants.

1 Speech system restricted. Consonants limited to nasals and/or approximants. May have a predominance of one sound only, including a glottal pattern.

2 Able to use 2 or more consonants in single words and structured activities. Poor transfer to sentence level and no generalization.

3 Mostly clear articulation. One or more articulation errors which require therapy at this time. Articulation not consistent in spontaneous speech, especially when tired or excited.

4 Persistent minor errors. May have persistent minor errors (e.g., anterior cleft speech errors or minor developmental errors) not affecting intelligibility and not requiring therapy at this time.

5 Age-appropriate articulation.

Activity

0 Completely unintelligible to familiar and non-familiar listeners. Unable to make recognizable words.

1 Partially intelligible to familiar listeners in known context. Limited to a few recognizable words. Communication partner bears the burden of the responsibility.

2 Intelligible to familiar listeners in context. Non-familiar listeners able to understand occasional words.

3 Usually intelligible to familiar listeners in and out of context. Non-familiar listeners able to understand in context. Generally difficult to understand when excited or talking quickly.

4 Minor problems. Only occasionally unintelligible to everyone.

5 Fully intelligible at an age-appropriate level to familiar and non-familiar listeners alike.

Participation

0 Profound difficulties in participating. Unable to participate in any social/educational/family role. No social integration.

1 Very severe difficulties in participating. Very little confidence. Doesn't speak outside of home environment. Socially isolated.

2 Severe difficulties in participating. Some self-confidence. Needs a lot of support to join in.

3 Moderate difficulties in participating. Will mix socially in certain environments. Able to integrate socially but needs encouragement.

4 Mild difficulties in participating. Willing to mix socially in most environments, with occasional difficulties in some situations. Occasionally seeks out assistance with some social activities.

5 No difficulties in participating. Fully confident in social, family and educational context.

Wellbeing

0 Profound distress. Always severely withdrawn, frustrated or depressed. Unable to express or control emotions appropriately.

1 Very severe distress . Very frequent episodes of upset /frustration/anger/embarrassment/ withdrawal. Becomes concerned easily; requires frequent support; loses emotional control easily.

2 Severe distress. Frequent episodes of upset/frustration/anger/embarrassment/ withdrawal. Emotional encouragement and support required, especially in unfamiliar situations.

3 Moderate distress. Occasional episodes of upset/frustration/anger/embarrassment/ withdrawal.. Emotionally dependent on some occasions. Vulnerable to changes in routine.

4 Mild distress or upset/frustration/anger/embarrassment/withdrawal. Generally well adjusted with only occasional emotional support required.

5 No distress. Accepts and understands own limitations, coping emotionally in most situations as appropriate for age.

Acknowledgement: Stephanie van Eeden, Marion Hall, Sonia McVay, Jacqueline Miller, Caroline Smith and Samantha Marshman, Newcastle Cleft Palate Team.

62 Vocal Tract Discomfort

Scale in development
Identify descriptor that is 'best fit'. The patient/client/student does not have to have each feature mentioned. Use 0.5 to indicate if patient/client/student is slightly better or worse than a descriptor. Consider as appropriate for age gender and culture.

Impairment

0 Extremely severe and/or constant symptom(s) including burning, tightness, dryness, ache, tickle, soreness, irritation and/or lump in throat sensation.

1 Severe and/or highly frequent symptom(s) as above.

2 Severe/moderate and/or frequent symptom(s) as above.

3 Moderate and/or regular symptom(s) as above.

4 Mild and/or intermittent/occasional symptom(s) as above.

5 No vocal tract discomfort.

Activity

0 Vocal tract discomfort consistently preventing all voice use or swallowing.

1 Vocal tract discomfort frequently preventing significant voice use or swallowing.

2 Vocal tract discomfort often preventing many aspects of voice use or swallowing.

3 Vocal tract discomfort sometimes disrupting voice use or swallowing.

4 Vocal tract discomfort occasionally disrupting voice use or swallowing.

5 No disruption of voice or swallowing.

Participation

0 No autonomy, isolated, no social/family life.

1 Very limited choices, contact mainly with professionals, no social or family role, little control over life.

2 Some integration, value and autonomy in one setting.

3 Integrated, valued and autonomous in limited number of settings.

4 Occasionally some restriction in autonomy, integration or role.

5 Integrated, valued, occupies appropriate role.

Wellbeing/Distress (client/carer)

0 Severe constant: High and constant levels of distress/upset/concern/frustration/ anger/embarrassment/withdrawal/severe depression/apathy. Unable to express or control emotions appropriately.

1 Frequently severe: Moderate distress/upset/concern/frustration/anger/embarrassment/ withdrawal/severe depression/apathy. Becomes concerned easily, requires constant reassurance/support, needs clear/tight limits and structure, loses emotional control easily.

2 Moderate consistent: Distress/upset/concern/frustration/anger/embarrassment/ withdrawal/severe depression/apathy in unfamiliar situations, frequent emotional encouragement and support required.

3 Moderate frequent: Distress/upset/concern/frustration/anger/embarrassment/ withdrawal/severe depression/apathy. Controls emotions with assistance, emotionally dependent on some occasions, vulnerable to changes in routine, etc., spontaneously uses methods to assist emotional control.

4 Mild occasional: Distress/upset/concern/frustration/anger/embarrassment/withdrawal/ severe depression/apathy. Able to control feelings in most situations, generally well adjusted/stable (most of the time/most situations), occasional emotional support/ encouragement needed

5 Not inappropriate: Distress/upset/concern/frustration/anger/embarrassment/ withdrawal/severe depression/apathy. Well adjusted, stable and able to cope emotionally with most situations, good insight, accepts and understands own limitations

Acknowledgement: Developed by Jenny Evans, Medway Community Healthcare, with the assistance of others.

63 Attention Deficit Hyperactivity Disorder

Scale in development
The individual does not have to have each feature mentioned in the descriptor. It is a best fit description, i.e,. does this description fit the individual better than the other one. Use 0.5 to indicate if the individual is slightly better or worse than the descriptor.

Impairment

0 Profound ADHD. Cannot concentrate on even simple task. Constantly distracted by environmental objects and noises. Constantly physically restless. Frequently loses temper. Avoids any interaction which requires attention. Makes choices and decisions without considering options and consequences. Continually spontaneous in action and reaction.

1 Severe/moderate ADHD. Very occasional ability to concentrate on a task of interest. May not be distracted for a short period of time when involved in task of interest. Avoids interaction which requires particular level of attention. Very occasional periods when not physically restless.

2 Moderate ADHD. Ability to concentrate/attend to a task is highly variable and unpredictable. Short periods of good concentration and attention. Focus on task is not necessarily helped by reduced environmental distraction.

3 Moderate/mild ADHD. Periods when it is difficult to concentrate or attend to a task. Some environments or times of the day are consistently difficult. Short periods of muscular restlessness. Focus on task is helped by reduced environmental distraction.

4 Mild ADHD. Occasional difficulties concentrating particularly when environment is distracting. Has some awareness of difficulty which causes frustration and irritation. Can make extra effort to concentrate when encouraged to do so. Generally able to follow activity or topics that require some effort.

5 Able to concentrate on tasks appropriate for age. Not easily distracted. Can interact and do tasks which require age-appropriate attention

Activity

0 No regard for impact of behaviour on others. No regard for personal safety or safety of others. Totally disruptive for known cooperative behaviour. Requires consistent vigilant supervision. Unable to communicate consistently or effectively. Severe challenging behaviour which may include self-harm, aggression.

1 Occasional regard as to impact of behaviour on others. Tendency to be disruptive and uncooperative. Requires high level of assistance and supervision in all tasks. Occasionally able to communicate effectively and appropriately in one context when attention is not demanded. Frequent periods of inappropriate challenging behaviour which may include self-harm and aggression.

2 Some regard of impact of behaviour on others. Can cooperate but requires high level of assistance, encouragement and supervision in most tasks. Some limited functional communication but tends to switch topic and lose the thread of conversation easily, particularly when distracted. Able to make basic needs known and follow simple instructions out of context. Communicates better in familiar surroundings.

3 Responds to encouragement and instruction regarding impact of behaviour on others. Needs and responds to assistance in organizing tasks and behaviours in some contexts. Consistently able to communicate effectively and appropriately in more than one context but not in all situations. Able to follow most simple and everyday conversations in context; can communicate equally well with familiar people and strangers in some unfamiliar as well as familiar settings but this is not consistent. Needs fewer cues and assistance overall. Self regulates in most situations. Tends to lose concentration required for physical tasks and conversation particularly when tired or in unfamiliar surroundings.

4 Requires some advice, support and reminder of strategies in order to manage behaviour and engage with tasks and conversation. Mostly resilient to distraction and physical restlessness but personal effort is required. Fully aware of impact of behaviour on others. Communication ability is normal in the majority of contexts.

5 Independence in all activities. Appropriate engagement with activities.

Participation

0 Unable to fulfil any relationship roles. Not involved in decision making/lacks motivation or responsibility/no investment in self or others/isolates self/lacks trust.

1 Low self-confidence/poor self esteem. Wary of establishing individual relationships. Unable to take responsibility for self. Seeks to avoid making decisions pertaining to self.

2 Some self-confidence/some social interaction. Able to tolerate some group situations, although does not invest self into these. Still prefers to be alone and defer responsibility for decision making.

3 Some self-confidence, autonomy emerging. More social integration seen through own volition. Beginning to take some decisions with support. Shows more investment in self and willingness to trust others.

4 Mostly confident/occasional difficulties in interaction. Integrating more readily in variety of situations. Shows autonomy when making most decisions. More able to trust a range of people. On occasion does not fulfil relationship potential.

5 Achieving relationship roles/potential/autonomous.

Wellbeing/Distress (client/carer)

0 Severe constant: High and constant levels of distress/upset/concern/frustration/anger/embarrassment/withdrawal/severe depression/apathy. Unable to express or control emotion appropriately.

1 Frequently severe: Moderate distress/upset/concern/frustration/anger/embarrassment/withdrawal/severe depression/apathy. Becomes concerned easily, requires constant reassurance/support, needs clear/tight limits and structure, loses emotional control easily.

2 Moderate consistent: Distress/upset/concern/frustration/anger/embarrassment/withdrawal/severe depression/apathy in unfamiliar situations. Frequent emotional encouragement and support required.

3 Moderate frequent: Distress/upset/concern/frustration/anger/embarrassment/withdrawal/severe depression/apathy. Controls emotions with assistance, emotionally dependent on some occasions, vulnerable to change in routine, etc., spontaneously uses methods to assist emotional control.

4 Mild occasional: Distress/upset/concern/frustration/anger/embarrassment/withdrawal/severe depression/apathy. Able to control feelings in most situations, generally well adjusted/stable (most of the time/most situations), occasional emotional support/encouragement needed.

5 Not inappropriate: Distress/upset/concern/frustration/anger/embarrassment/withdrawal/severe depression/apathy. Well adjusted, stable and able to cope emotionally with most situations, good insight, accepts and understands own limitations.

Acknowledgement: Camilla Sanossian-East in collaboration with Pam Enderby.

64 Auditory Impairment/Deafness/Partially Hearing

Scale in development
Identify descriptor that is 'best fit'. The patient/client/student does not have to have each feature mentioned. Use 0.5 to indicate if patient/client/student is slightly better or worse than a descriptor and as appropriate to age.

Impairment

0 Profound hearing loss. Unable to hear any speech or environmental sounds.

1 Severe hearing loss. Can perceive very restricted range of environmental and speech sounds.

2 Severe/moderate hearing loss. Requires attention to perceive a limited range of speech and environmental sounds.

3 Moderate hearing loss. Can hear a range of speech and environmental sounds.

4 Mild hearing loss. Unable to hear some specific frequencies; can hear most speech and environmental sounds.

5 Normal hearing.

Activity 1 Communication

0 No functional communication. Unable to communicate needs or preferences. Needs familiar or highly-trained people to identify possible indications of needs or preferences.

1 Limited functional communication with familiar people who are trained in meeting their communication needs. Adapted environments or communication modes required. Minimal communication with high levels of assistance.

2 Developing functional communication with familiar people. Able to make needs and preferences known approximately 50% of the time with medium levels of assistance. Communication breakdowns are frequent and difficulties with communication repair.

3 Consistent level of general functional communication with trained or familiar people. Able to make requests, comments and ask questions. Communication breakdowns continue to occur, especially if context is less familiar. Reliance on communication partner to facilitate communication repair.

4 Able to communicate effectively in most situations. May continue to present with mild difficulties when communicating complex ideas or with unfamiliar people. Attempts to repair communication breakdown.

5 Consistent effective communication.

Activity 2 Amplification use

0 No use of amplification.

1 Limited use of amplification. Resists wearing aid/cochlear implant. Frequently avoids aids or implants being put on as well as pulling them off. Needs high level of distraction to wear aids/implants for short periods of time.

2 Wears aids/implants for longer periods of time. Needs distraction initially to put device on but then wears them for prolonged time without support. Unable to indicate fault with device.

3 Wears aids/implants consistently in some environments. Does not wear devices in all communication settings, e.g., home. Not consistently or delayed in indicating fault with device.

4 Consistent user of hearing aids/implants. Will request device. Needs support to indicate a fault with device.

5 Consistent user of hearing aids/implants. Can indicate if there are faults with device. Able to maintain aids independently or able to indicate if further support is required.

Participation

0 No control over their environment or events/activities they are part of. Not involved in any decision making. Not integrated into their social settings or activities.

1 Some control over their environment or activities they are part of. Able to make some basic decisions. Low self-confidence/poor self-esteem/socially isolated. Unable to achieve potential in identified situations.

2 Able to control and make decisions in familiar activities, environments or with familiar people. Can integrate into social settings or activities with a high level of support. Some self-confidence in familiar situations.

3 Confidence and decision making becoming more secure. Limited social integration or participation achieved with support. Needs encouragement to achieve potential in more challenging situations.

4 Mostly confident and can make decisions in most situations. Occasional difficulties integrating into a social setting or activity, but needs minimal support to overcome this. May experience some difficulties achieving potential in challenging situations.

5 Able to participate in all social settings and activities. Is able to make decisions and exert control over all aspects of their life. Achieves potential in all areas.

Wellbeing/Distress (client/carer)

0 Severe constant: High and constant levels of distress/upset/concern/frustration/anger/embarrassment/withdrawal/severe depression/apathy. Unable to express or control emotions appropriately in all situations.

1 Frequently severe: Moderate levels of distress/upset/concern/frustration/anger/embarrassment/withdrawal/severe depression/apathy. Becomes concerned or agitated easily. Requires constant reassurance or support. Needs clear boundaries and structure. Loses emotional control easily.

2 Moderate consistent: Distress/upset/concern/frustration/anger/embarrassment/withdrawal/severe depression/apathy in unfamiliar situations. Frequent emotional encouragement and support required.

3 Moderate frequent: Controls emotions on some occasions with support. Vulnerable to change in routine. Able to use methods to assist emotional control.

4 Mild occasional: Able to control feelings in most situations. Generally emotionally stable or well adjusted. Occasionally requires emotional support/encouragement.

5 Not inappropriate: Well adjusted, stable and able to cope emotionally with most situations. Good insight into their own emotions. Accepts and understands their limitations/needs.

Acknowledgement: Lisa Nash in collaboration with Pam Enderby.

65 Infant Pre-feeding Skills

Scale in development
Identify descriptor that is 'best fit'. The patient/client/student does not have to have each feature mentioned. Use 0.5 to indicate if patient/client/student is slightly better or worse than a descriptor. Consider as appropriate for age gender and culture.

Impairment

0 Absent. No evidence of the presence of pre-feeding skills, e.g., no non-nutritive suck (NNS), rooting, or cueing behaviours. May or may not be related to state of alertness.

1 Severe. Inconsistent **and** disorganized/dysfunctional/immature pre-feeding skills. May or may not be related to state of alertness.

2 Severe/moderate. One pre-feeding skill reliably present only **but** remains disorganized/dysfunctional/immature. May or may not be related to state of alertness.

3 Moderate. More than one element of pre-feeding skills reliably present **but** remains disorganized/dysfunctional/immature. May or may not be related to state of alertness.

4 Mild. Consistent pre-feeding skills present with occasional difficulties present in one element even when in optimum state of alertness, e.g., disorganized NNS.

5 Normal pre-feeding skills when in optimum state of alertness.

Activity

0 No opportunity. No evidence of MDT facilitation of pre-feeding skills development with parents/carer, e.g., no NNS, skin to skin, sensitive mouth care. All carried out by MDT only.

1 Limited opportunity. Minimal evidence of MDT facilitation of pre-feeding skills development with parents/carer. 10% carried out by parents/carer with experienced supervision.

2 Inconsistent opportunity. Inconsistent evidence of MDT facilitation of pre-feeding skills development with parents/carer. Less than 50% carried out by parents/carer with experienced supervision.

3 Supported opportunity. Consistent evidence of MDT facilitation of pre-feeding skills development with parents/carer. More than 50% carried out by parents/carer with experienced supervision.

4 Consistent opportunity. Consistent evidence of pre-feeding skills development opportunities with parents/carer. More than 90% carried out by parents/carer with occasional supervision.

5 Competent autonomous opportunity. Consistent evidence of pre-feeding skills development opportunities with parents/carer. All carried out by parent/carers. No supervision needed.

Participation

0 Unable to fulfil any social/educational/family role. Not involved in decision making/ no autonomy/no control over environment, no social integration.

1 Very limited choices. Contact mainly with professionals, no social or family role, little control over life, limited ability to make lifestyle choices, food choices, treatment options.

2 Some self-confidence/some social integration. Makes some decisions and influences control in familiar situations.

3 Some self-confidence; autonomy emerging. Makes decisions and has control of some aspects of life. Able to achieve some limited social integration/educational activities. Diffident over control over life. Needs encouragement to achieve potential.

4 Mostly confident. Occasional difficulties integrating or in fulfilling social/role activity. Participates in all appropriate decisions. May have difficulty in achieving potential in some situations occasionally.

5 Achieving potential. Autonomous and unrestricted. Able to fulfil social, educational and family role. Takes responsibility for own health.

Wellbeing/Distress (infant/carer)

0 Severe constant: High and constant levels of distress/upset/concern/frustration/ anger/embarrassment/withdrawal/severe depression/apathy. Unable to express or control emotions appropriately.

1 Frequently severe: Moderate distress/upset/concern/frustration/anger/embarrassment/ withdrawal/severe depression/apathy. Becomes concerned easily, requires constant reassurance/support, needs clear/tight limits and structure, loses emotional control easily.

2 Moderate consistent: Distress/upset/concern/frustration/anger/embarrassment/ withdrawal/severe depression/apathy in unfamiliar situations, frequent emotional encouragement and support required.

3 Moderate frequent: Distress/upset/concern/frustration/anger/embarrassment/ withdrawal/severe depression/apathy. Controls emotions with assistance, emotionally dependent on some occasions, vulnerable to change in routine, etc., spontaneously uses methods to assist emotional control.

4 Mild occasional: Distress/upset/concern/frustration/anger/embarrassment/withdrawal/ severe depression/apathy. Able to control feelings in most situations, generally well adjusted/stable (most of the time/most situations), occasional emotional support/ encouragement needed.

5 Not inappropriate: Distress/upset/concern/frustration/anger/embarrassment/ withdrawal/severe depression/apathy. Well adjusted, stable and able to cope emotionally.

Acknowledgement: M Peck and A Connolly (2018), Royal London Children's Hospital.

66 Social Communication Difficulty

Scale in development
Identify descriptor that is 'best fit'. The patient/client/student does not have to have each feature mentioned. Use 0.5 to indicate if patient/client/student is slightly better or worse than a descriptor and as appropriate to age.

Impairment

0 No engagement with others. No eye contact. Mute or restricted to a small number of words/phrases/sounds sometimes used repetitively with no communicative intent. Does not respond to stimulation appropriately. Does not distinguish between positive and negative vocal tones. Not interested/doesn't understand emotions of others even if clearly expressed. Will not be directed by adult. Reacts negatively to change. Extremely distressed when not in familiar situations or surroundings. No appropriate use of verbal or nonverbal language in communication with others.

1 Severe impairment in multiple areas including verbal communication, nonverbal communication, social interaction. Some occasional and limited communicative intent, e.g., basic verbal or nonverbal requests to meet some of own needs. Lacks appropriate use of relevant language (verbal and nonverbal) in communication with others. Unaware of turn taking. Very occasional interest/response to other people. Mostly reacts negatively to change. Becomes distressed when out of routine. Can only be directed by adult very occasionally.

2 Moderate/severe impairment. Has reasonable but limited vocabulary and use of communicative sounds but verbal and nonverbal communication deficits are obvious to all. Use of verbal and nonverbal language is frequently socially inappropriate with stilted social interaction and limited understanding of social rules. Shows some limited but appropriate use of relevant language in communication with others in specific settings. Does not turn-take in play or communication. Can be directed by adult in some situations. Can tolerate some change in surroundings and routines but needs support/preparation.

3 Moderate impairment. Abnormal or unusual speaking style, voice and/or manner of speech which may occasionally be repetitive. Nonverbal communication deficits are obvious to a non-skilled observer, e.g., abnormal posture, use of hand gestures, limited facial expression, limited eye contact. Some limited use of appropriate and relevant language in communication with others in learned social settings. Turn-taking generally present in known situations/settings. Formulaic social interactions. Variability in following social rules. Regularly accepts direction from familiar adults in familiar surroundings. Can tolerate some change in surroundings and routines but prefers familiar surroundings and routines.

4 Slight impairment. Difficulties in communication are subtle. Able to use appropriate and relevant verbal and nonverbal language in communication with others but this can break down on occasions. Able to take turns with familiar partners. May have monotonous voice, pedantic speech or other idiosyncrasies. Rigid thinking style, perhaps evidenced by over-literal interpretations or inability to understand idioms, sarcasm and humour, etc. Difficulty with empathy. Social rules are learned formulaically but not necessarily natural or automatic. Can manage in a range of surroundings and with changes in routine.

5 No impairment. Good social communication.

Activity

0 Dependent for all the functional tasks. Unable to meet basic self-care needs. Unable to communicate effectively in any way. Frequently distressed. Self-directed, does not engage in any pretend play. Repetitive behaviours. Likely to exhibit challenging behaviours which can be extreme.

1 Dependent for most tasks but occasional cooperation. Able to meet some self-care needs. Limited communication through verbal or nonverbal means which can be interpreted by those familiar with the individual. Inconsistent or inappropriate eye contact and nonverbal communication. Engages in repetitive, limited pretend play. Very limited understanding of speech, nonverbal communication and the emotions of others. Likely to have repetitive, purposeless and challenging behaviours which can be extreme in new situations. Follows own interests.

2 Needs verbal/physical prompts and support/encouragement to initiate/undertake most tasks. Limited understanding of speech, nonverbal communication and emotions of others. Able to engage in basic communication related to the present. Comfortable with repetition. Will be able to comprehend limited and obvious nonverbal cues (e.g,. can tell that someone is upset if they are crying) but unable to understand more subtle nonverbal cues. May have repetitive, purposeless behaviours and mannerisms in some situations. Need for routine, exhibits anxiety/anger in novel situations. Engages in some pretend play. Focuses on topics of interest to self, shows difficulties with topic maintenance.

3 Initiates appropriately but might need some support and encouragement to undertake less usual activities, particularly involving less familiar individuals. Mostly understands and responds appropriately in limited, familiar situation with familiar others. Difficulty in understanding and appropriately responding in less usual social situation or larger groups. Difficulty in appreciating the needs and emotions of others. Able to meet some self-care needs. Able to conduct a factual conversation related to the present but it may be stilted or one-sided. May have restricted range of interests. Engages in pretend play but this tends to be repetitive and limited in fantasy. Purposeless, repetitive behaviour is less prominent. Preference for topics of interest to self and difficulties with topic maintenance.

4 Able to manage most activities of daily living appropriate for age. Some misunderstandings of speech, nonverbal communication, situations and the emotions of others. Able to communicate effectively with familiar persons but may have difficulties with subtleties of verbal and nonverbal communication. Social interaction may be less natural with difficulties appreciating humour, sarcasm, irony. May be seen as 'different' by others, and may be unaware of indiscretions in social situations. A preference for routine. Able to sustain and maintain a topic with some support.

5 Communicates as appropriate for age in all situations.

Participation

0 Unable to fulfil any social/occupational/family role. No autonomy. No control and the environment. No social integration.

1 Low self-confidence/poor self-esteem/limited social integration/socially isolated. Unable to fulfil any educational/occupational role. No friends/acquaintances outside family/carers. Only able to engage in social activities with large amounts of support from carers.

2 Some degree of self-confidence and social integration beyond immediate family and carers. Fulfils some social/occupational/education or family role with support. Able to effect some decisions/control in familiar situations. Social life will be very limited.

3 Makes decisions and has control over some aspects of life. Able to engage with family/occupation/recreation/education system to some extent with appropriate adjustment and support. Has a few friends/acquaintances. Has some autonomy and control over life. Needs encouragement to achieve potential.

4 Autonomous in most or all activities. May have occasional difficulties integrating or in fulfilling social/role activity. May have difficulty in achieving potential in some situations on some occasions. May have restricted interests/pastimes.

5 Autonomous in all activities. Able to fill social, occupational and family role.

Wellbeing (client/carer)

0 High and constant levels of distress and problematic emotions, like frustration/elation anger, etc. May have severe depression and/or severe anxiety. May have severe apathy/social withdrawal. Likely to be unable to express or control emotions appropriately.

1 Severe levels of distress and problematic emotions. These are present all or nearly all of the time. Becomes distressed easily, requires constant reassurance/support, needs clear/tight limits and structure, loses emotional control easily.

2 Moderate to severe levels of distress and problematic emotions. Present most of the time. Frequent emotional support required.

3 Moderate levels of distress and problematic emotions. Occur frequently, more likely to occur in novel situations/changes in routine. Controls emotions with assistance, emotionally dependent on some occasions, but can use strategies to assist emotional control.

4 Mild levels of distress and problematic emotions. Not present all the time, likely only associated with novel situations or changes of routine. Able to control feelings in most situations, generally well adjusted/stable (most of the time/most situations), occasional emotional support needed.

5 Not inappropriate distress/upset/concern/frustration/anger/distress/embarrassment/ withdrawal/severe depression/apathy. Well adjusted, stable and able to cope emotionally with most situations, good insight, accepts and understands own limitations.

Acknowledgement: Alex John in collaboration with Pam Enderby.

67 Pragmatic Communication Disorder

Scale in development
Use this scale if the symptoms are not attributable to another medical or neurological condition or to low abilities in the domains of word structure and grammar, and are not better explained by autistic spectrum disorder, intellectual disability (intellectual developmental disorder), global developmental delay, or another mental disorder. Identify descriptor that is 'best fit'. The patient/client/student does not have to have each feature mentioned. Use 0.5 to indicate if patient/client/student is slightly better or worse than a descriptor and as appropriate to age.

Impairment

0 Profound. Impairment and persistent difficulties in the social use of verbal and nonverbal language, in using communication for social purposes including any greeting and sharing of information. Unable to change communication to match the context or the needs of the listener, the setting or situation. Unable to follow rules of conversation and narrative, taking turns in conversation, maintaining a topic, rephrasing/recasting when misunderstood. Does not use verbal and nonverbal signals to regulate interaction. Unable to understand what is not explicitly stated, make inferences and nonliteral or ambiguous meaning of language, including idioms, humour, metaphors, multiple meanings that depend on the context for interpretation.

1 Severe and persistent difficulties in the social use of verbal and nonverbal language in using communication for social purposes including greeting and sharing information in a manner that is appropriate for the social context. Difficulty in the ability to change communication to match the context or the needs of the listener, the setting or situation. Unable to follow rules of conversation and narrative, including inability to take turns in conversation, in maintaining a topic, rephrasing/recasting when misunderstood, understanding how to use verbal and nonverbal signals to regulate interaction. Unable to understand what is not explicitly stated, inferences and nonliteral or ambiguous meaning of language, including idioms, humour, metaphors, multiple meanings that depend on the context for interpretation.

2 Severe/moderate. Frequently has difficulty in the social use of verbal and nonverbal language in using communication for social purposes including greeting and sharing information in a manner that is appropriate for the social context. However, can very occasionally and in some settings perform some limited communication appropriately. Frequently has difficulty in changing communication to match the context or the needs of the listener, the setting or situation. Has difficulty with following rules of conversation and narrative, including taking turns in conversation, maintaining a topic, rephrasing/recasting when misunderstood, understanding how to use verbal and nonverbal signals to regulate interaction. Frequently misunderstands what is not explicitly stated, making inferences and nonliteral or ambiguous meaning of language, including idioms, humour, metaphors, multiple meanings that depend on the context for interpretation.

3 Moderate. Has some difficulty in the social use of verbal and nonverbal language in using communication for social purposes including greeting and sharing information in a manner that is appropriate for the social context particularly in less usual situations and contexts. However, has some ability to change communication to match the context or the needs of the listener, the setting or situation. Able to follow learned rules of conversation and narrative in known settings, learning to taking turns in conversation in familiar settings, able to maintain a topic for a short time when familiar with the topic, some emergence of rephrasing/recasting when misunderstood, some understanding of how to use verbal and nonverbal signals to regulate interaction. Some difficulties understanding what is not explicitly stated, making inferences and nonliteral or ambiguous meaning of language, including idioms, humour, metaphors, multiple meanings that depend on the context for interpretation particularly in new situations or with new communication partners.

4 Occasional difficulty in the social use of verbal and nonverbal language in using communication for social purposes including sharing information in a manner that is appropriate for the social context. Occasional difficulties in ability to change communication to match the context or the needs of the listener, the setting or situation. Occasional difficulties following rules of conversation and narrative, includes difficulties in taking turns in conversation, in maintaining a topic, rephrasing/recasting when misunderstood, understanding how to use verbal and nonverbal signals to regulate interaction. Occasional difficulties understanding what is not explicitly stated, making inferences and nonliteral or ambiguous meaning of language, including idioms, humour, metaphors, multiple meanings that depend on the context for interpretation. These difficulties are particularly obvious when in new contexts or when unable to concentrate.

5 No difficulty with social communication. Able to use verbal and nonverbal language in communication for social purposes including greeting and sharing information in a manner that is appropriate for the social context.

Activity

0 No independent functional communication. Lacks effective communication. Communication is affected by very limited understanding of the situational context; does not provide a context for listener understanding. Communication is never effective due to a lack of perspective to take in communicative situations, problem solving or predicting. Disregards communication partner.

1 Limited functional communication, some verbal and nonverbal communication can be interpreted by those familiar with the individual. Communication is affected by very limited understanding of situational context; limited context provided for listener understanding. Extremely limited perspective taking in communicative situations; extremely limited problem solving and ability to predict which affects communication. Unable to respond to assistance of communication partner

2 Some functional communication, verbal and nonverbal communication can be interpreted reliably by those familiar with the individual in familiar contexts. Communication is affected by very limited understanding of unfamiliar and novel situational context; occasionally context is provided for listener understanding. Some limited perspective in communicative situations; some limited problem solving and ability to predict which affects/assists communication with others. Occasionally responds to assistance of communication partner

3 Functional communication with familiar communication partners. Effectiveness of communication can be affected by limitations in ability to understand unfamiliar and novel situational contexts; a familiar listener can support provision of context to support understanding. Able to use some perspective in familiar situations and with familiar communication partners; achieving some problem solving or predicting when communicating when given cues and strategies. Responds to assistance of communication partner.

4 Functional communication, verbal and nonverbal communication with unfamiliar communication partners. Understands most unfamiliar and novel situational contexts; occasionally needs a familiar listener to support provision of context to support understanding. Able to use perspective taking in most situations and with unfamiliar communication partners; frequently achieves problem solving or predicting when communicating with others. Communication occasionally derailed but can self-correct.

5 Uses effective verbal and nonverbal communication in all settings. Understands unfamiliar and novel situational contexts. Able to use perspective taking in situations with communication partners; uses problem solving and predicting when communicating with others.

Participation

0 Unable to fulfil any social/occupational/family role. No autonomy. No control over the environment. No social integration. Profound difficulties in forming social relationships which impacts on social life, in undertaking academic work or in undertaking occupations that require social communication skills.

1 Low self-confidence/poor self-esteem/limited social integration/socially isolated. Unable to fulfil any educational/occupational role. No friends/acquaintances outside family/carers. Only able to engage in social activities with large amounts of support from carers.

2 Some degree of self-confidence and social integration beyond immediate family and carers. Fulfils some social/occupational/education/family role with support. Able to effect some decisions/control in familiar situations. Social life very limited.

3 Makes decisions and has control over some aspects of life. Able to engage with family/ occupation/recreation/education system to some extent with appropriate adjustment and support. Has a few friends/acquaintances. Has some autonomy and control over life. Needs encouragement to achieve potential.

4 Autonomous in most or all activities. May have occasional difficulties integrating or in fulfilling social/role activity. May have difficulty in achieving potential in some situations on some occasions. May have restricted interests/pastimes.

5 Autonomous in all activities. Able to fill social, occupational and family role.

Wellbeing/Distress (client/carer)

0 High and constant levels of distress and problematic emotions, like frustration/elation/ anger, etc. May have severe depression and/or severe anxiety. May have severe apathy/ social withdrawal. Likely to be unable to express or control emotions appropriately.

1 Severe levels of distress and problematic emotions. These are present all or nearly all of the time. Becomes distressed easily, requires constant reassurance/support, needs clear/tight limits and structure, loses emotional control easily.

2 Moderate to severe levels of distress and problematic emotions present most of the time. Frequent emotional support required.

3 Moderate levels of distress and problematic emotions. Occur frequently, more likely to occur in novel situations/changes in routine. Controls emotions with assistance, emotionally dependent on some occasions, but can use strategies to assist emotional control.

4 Mild levels of distress and problematic emotions. Not present all the time, likely only associated with novel situations or changes of routine. Able to control feelings in most situations, generally well adjusted/stable (most of the time/most situations), occasional emotional support needed.

5 Not inappropriate: Distress/upset/concern/frustration/anger/embarrassment/ withdrawal/severe depression or apathy. Well adjusted, stable and able to cope emotionally with most situations, good insight, accepts and understands own limitations.

Acknowledgement Alexandra John

68 Articulation Disorder

Scale in development
The individual does not have to have each feature mentioned in the descriptor. It is a best fit description, i.e., does this description fit the individual better than the other one. Use 0.5 to indicate if the individual is slightly better or worse than the descriptor. Consider as appropriate for age.

Impairment

0 Profound. Limited sound system; few recognizable consonants articulated or imitated correctly and consistently; few vowel sounds articulated or imitated correctly and consistently; significant difficulty with resonance impacting on all sounds

1 Severe. Less than 50% of consonants expected at their age articulated correctly. Some consistent consonant-vowel or vowel-consonant combinations articulated or imitated correctly and consistently; limited range of vowel sounds articulated or imitated correctly and consistently; significant difficulty with resonance impacting on majority of sounds.

2 Severe/Moderate Less than 65% of the consonants expected at their age articulated correctly; some consonant-vowel-consonant combinations articulated or imitated correctly and consistently; multiple vowel errors evident; frequent difficulties with resonance impacting on a range of sounds.

3 Moderate. 65-84% of the consonants expected at their age articulated correctly; beginning to use more complex sound combinations, e.g., consonant-vowel-consonant-consonant correctly and consistently; some vowel errors evident particularly with diphthongs; resonance difficulties impacting a type of sound, e.g., fricatives; disordered articulation of one sound or a type of sounds, e.g., lateral 's', active nasal fricatives.

4 Mild. 85% of the consonants expected at their age articulated correctly; vowel sounds articulated accurately; difficulty with multisyllabic words; no resonance difficulties; speech immaturities, e.g., incorrect interdental articulation.

5 Age-appropriate articulation. Normal resonance.

Activity

0 Completely unintelligible to familiar and non-familiar listeners.

1 Not intelligible to non-familiar listeners. Partly intelligible to familiar listeners in known context; communication partner bears the burden of the responsibility.

2 Intelligible to familiar listeners in context; partly intelligible in context with non-familiar listeners. Unintelligible in connected speech.

3 Usually intelligible to familiar listeners in and out of context; variable intelligibility in context with non-familiar listeners; free, spontaneous speech can be unintelligible.

4 Minor problems but intelligible to everyone; occasionally loses intelligibility, for example when excited or speaking against noise, etc.

5 Intelligible at age-appropriate level to familiar listeners and non-familiar listeners.

Participation

0 Unable to fulfil any social/educational/family role. Not involved in decision-making, no autonomy, no control over environment, no social integration.

1 Low self-confidence, poor self-esteem, limited social integration, socially isolated, contributes to some basic and limited decisions. Cannot achieve potential in any situation.

2 Some self-confidence, some social integration, makes some decisions and influences control in familiar situations.

3 Some self-confidence; autonomy emerging. Makes decisions and has control of some aspects of life. Able to achieve some limited social integration/educational activities. Diffident over control over life. Needs encouragement to achieve potential.

4 Mostly confident. Occasional difficulties in integrating or in fulfilling social/role activity. Participates in all appropriate decisions. May have difficulty in achieving potential in some situations occasionally.

5 Achieving potential. Autonomous and unrestricted. Able to fulfil social, educational and family role.

Wellbeing/Distress

0 Severe constant: High and constant levels of distress/upset/concern/frustration/anger/embarrassment/withdrawal/severe depression/apathy. Unable to express or control emotions appropriately.

1 Frequently severe: Moderate distress/upset/concern/frustration/anger/embarrassment/withdrawal/severe depression/apathy. Becomes concerned easily, requires constant reassurance/support, needs clear/tight limits and structure, loses emotional control easily.

2 Moderate consistent: Distress/upset/concern/frustration/anger/embarrassment/withdrawal/ severe depression/apathy in unfamiliar situations. Frequent emotional encouragement and support required.

3 Moderate frequent: Distress/upset/concern/frustration/anger/embarrassment/ withdrawal/severe depression/apathy. Controls emotions with assistance, emotionally dependent on some occasions, vulnerable to change in routine, etc., spontaneously uses methods to assist emotional control.

4 Mild occasional: Distress/upset/concern/frustration/anger/embarrassment/withdrawal/ severe depression/apathy. Able to control feelings in most situations, generally well adjusted/stable (most of the time/most situations), occasional emotional support/ encouragement needed.

5 Not inappropriate: Distress/upset/concern/frustration/anger/embarrassment/ withdrawal/severe depression/apathy. Well adjusted, stable and able to cope emotionally with most situations, good insight, accepts and understands own limitations.

Acknowledgement: Developed by Rachel Brown and Nicola Cuthbert-Brown (Surrey County Council SLT Service)

Accompanying Scales Additional to TOMs

The following scales have been developed by practitioners to provide additional information/context alongside the *Therapy Outcome Measures*. The authors/instigators have generously agreed to their inclusion in this User Guide.

1 Practitioner Confidence Questionnaire

(Shown opposite)

Objective:
To identify confidence and change in confidence in teachers following training or working with a speech and language therapist when the focus of the training is to improve participation in learning.

This form will be used to plan support for your school. It will be used by the speech and language therapist and may be shared with the school's lead practitioner but will not be shared more widely.

Developed by: The Communication & Language Team, Hampshire County Council. Accompanying scale for Therapy Outcome Measure in line with principles detailed in: Enderby, P. & John A. (2015). *Therapy Outcome Measures for Rehabilitation Professionals*, 3rd ed. Guildford: J&R Press.

Name of practitioner:	School:
Job role:	Date completed:

Rate your confidence in the areas listed below, where:
1 = Not at all Confident   6 = Extremely Confident

How confident are you in:	1	2	3	4	5	6
Knowledge of typical speech, language and communication development.						
Understanding the links between emotional development and speech, language and communication.						
Knowing how factors in the environment can impact on children's speech, language and communication development.						
Identifying children with speech, language and communication needs.						
Adapting the level of your language for individual children.						
Explicitly teaching vocabulary to children (knowing what words to teach and how best to teach them).						
Using the outdoor environment to support speech, language and communication development.						
Supporting children who are delayed with their language skills.						
Supporting children who are learning English as an additional language with their language development.						
Supporting children with specific communication needs, e.g., those accessing speech therapy, or with identified conditions like Autism.						
Knowing which children need a referral to speech and language therapy						
Enhancing language learning across all curriculum areas .						
Talking to parents about their child's speech, language and communication strengths and needs.						
Giving parents strategies and advice to support their child's speech, language and communication development.						
Total in each column						
Overall Confidence Score						

2 Feeding/Mealtime Enjoyment for Babies and Young Children with Dysphagia

Objective:
To reflect changes in mealtime behaviour in babies and children during feeding/mealtimes.

Feeding/Mealtime Enjoyment (if applicable)

0 Consistently shows high levels of distress (e.g., crying, gagging, behavioural stress cues) in response to touch to the face/mouth.

1 Consistently shows distress/refusal/avoidance/behavioural stress cues in response to feeding attempts. Sometimes tolerates touch to the face/mouth and tasters.

2 Occasionally shows enjoyment of feeding/eating/drinking but usually also shows distress/refusal/avoidance/behavioural stress cues in response to feeding attempts/mealtimes.

3 Sometimes shows enjoyment of feeding/eating/drinking/oral stimulation. Sometimes shows distress/refusal/avoidance/behavioural stress cues in response to feeding attempts/mealtimes.

4 Usually shows enjoyment of feeding/eating/drinking/oral stimulation. Occasionally shows distress at feed/meal times.

5 Enjoys feeding/eating/drinking/oral stimulation. No signs of distress at feed/meal times.

Acknowledgement: Bev Curtis, Cardiff and Vale University Health Board. Accompanying scale for Therapy Outcome Measure in line with principles detailed in: Enderby P. & John A. (2015). *Therapy Outcome Measures for Rehabilitation Professionals*, 3rd ed. Guildford: J&R Press.

3 Carer Confidence Scale

Objective:
To identify change in confidence in carers following training/support from a therapist.

Therapy Outcome Measure Additional Scale Carer Confidence	Confident	
I am confident that I understand and **I know how to help in all situations**.	5	🙂
I am mostly confident that I understand but have occasional difficulties. **I mostly know how to help.**	4.5 4	🙂
I am fairly confident that I understand what is helpful and know how to try different things but have some doubts. **I usually know how to help.**	3.5 3	😐
I have some confidence that I understand what to do but I have frequent doubts. **I sometimes know how to help**.	2.5 2	😐
I have a little confidence but often worry that I am not doing things right. **I frequently feel at a loss as to how to help.**	1.5 1	🙁
I am not confident that I understand what to do. **I don't know how to help.**	0.5 0	🙁
	No Confidence	

Acknowledgement: Bev Curtis, Cardiff and Vale University Health Board
Pam Enderby, Alex John, April 2017
Jennie Corkwood, January 2019

4 Support for Client: Environmental Controls Services

Objective: *To reflect context of support for the client using technology.*

Support

Note: 'Device' refers to any piece of assistive technology which has been prescribed or been given access to (e.g., environmental controller, computer, mobile phone).

0 No support. Client has no support in any of the environments where they use their device. Client has no one who understands how to use their device in any of their environments. No one has been identified that can support with initial familiarization with the device, ongoing training and settings updates (if applicable) to the device.

1 Limited support. Client has limited, inconsistent support in the environments where they use their device. Client is provided with few opportunities to use their device in their environment. Client has infrequent support from someone who understands how to use the basic features of the device. Client has limited, inconsistent support from someone who can help with initial familiarization with the device, ongoing training and settings updates (if applicable) to the device.

2 Inconsistent/inadequate support. Client has inconsistent/inadequate support in the environments where they use their device. Client has a small number of opportunities to use their device in their environment. Client sometimes has someone who will support them to use the device on a daily basis. Client has inconsistent/inadequate support from someone who understands how to use the basic features of the device. The client has some inconsistent/inadequate support from someone who can help with initial familiarization with the device, ongoing training and setting updates (if applicable) to the device.

3 Basic adequate, moderate support (bare minimum). Client has basic support in the environments where they use their device. Client has a satisfactory number of opportunities to use their device in their environment. Client has someone who will support them to use the device on a daily basis. Client has some consistent support from someone who understands how to use the basic features of the device. The client has adequate support from someone who can help with initial familiarization with the device, ongoing training and setting updates (if applicable) to the device.

4 Consistent support. Client usually has engaged support in all the environments they use their device. Client is consistently offered opportunities to use their device in their environment. Client has someone who will support them to use the device frequently on a daily basis. Client has consistent support from someone who understands how to use all of the features of the device. The client has ongoing support from someone who can help with initial familiarization with the device, ongoing training and setting updates (if applicable) to the device.

5 Excellent support. Client has full, engaged support in all of the environments they use their device. Client has full support from someone who will support them use the device constantly on a daily basis. Client is consistently given appropriate opportunities to use their device in their environment. Client has consistent support from multiple people who understand how to use all of the features of the device. The client has timely (proactive, pre-emptive) access to someone who is technically able and can provide support with initial familiarization with the device, ongoing training and setting updates (if applicable) to the device.

Acknowledgement: Graeme Marsh in collaboration with Environmental Controls Clinical Reference Group Environmental – Subgroup Working Party.

Accompanying scale for Therapy Outcome Measure in line with principles detailed in: Enderby P. & John A. (2015). *Therapy Outcome Measures for Rehabilitation Professionals*, 3rd ed. Guildford: J&R Press.

5 Supporting Equipment Use

Objective: to reflect context of support for the client using Augmentative and Alternative Communication (AAC).

0 No support. Client has no support in any of their environments/settings. Client has no one who has any knowledge of strategies for supporting communication (such as giving time, pausing, using aided language modelling). There is no recognition of the role of the communication partner. Client has no one who is aware of the individual's communication methods. Client has no opportunities to communicate. No one has been identified that can support with any coordination, maintenance and updating tasks related to the individual's communication methods (e.g., updating and sharing support documentation/information, editing paper based or electronic systems, setting and reviewing targets/goals). There is no one with whom support related advice and guidance can be provided or discussed.

1 Limited support. Client has limited support in their environments/settings or support is present in only one setting (where client accesses multiple settings) Client has limited number of communication partners who have knowledge of strategies for supporting communication (such as giving time, pausing, using aided language modelling). Poor recognition of the role of the communication partner. There are a limited range of communication partners who are aware of and able to support the individual's communication methods. Client is provided with limited/very few opportunities to communicate. There is poor coordination of and limited support with any maintenance and updating requirements of the individual's communication methods (e.g., updating and sharing support documentation/information, editing/updating paper based or electronic systems, setting and reviewing targets/goals).There is someone with whom support related advice and guidance can be provided or discussed but they are not able to respond to this or implement strategies.

2 Inconsistent /inadequate support. Client has inconsistent support in their environments/ settings or support is not present in all settings (where client accesses multiple settings). Client has a small number of communication partners who have knowledge of strategies for supporting communication (such as giving time, pausing, using aided language modelling). Few recognize of the role of the communication partner. There is a small number of communication partners who are aware of and able to support the individual's communication methods. Client is provided with an unsatisfactory number of opportunities to communicate. There is inadequate coordination of and support with any maintenance and updating requirements of the individual's communication methods (e.g. updating and sharing support documentation/information, editing/ updating paper based or electronic systems, setting and reviewing targets/goals). There is someone with whom support related advice and guidance can be provided or discussed but they are unlikely to respond to this or implement strategies.

3 Basic adequate, moderate support (bare minimum). Client has basic support in their environments/settings Client has an acceptable number of communication partners who have knowledge of strategies for supporting communication (such as giving time, pausing, using aided language modelling). There is some recognition of the role of the communication partner. There are some communication partners (in most or all environments) who are aware of and able to support the individual's communication methods. Client is provided with regular opportunities to communicate. There is some coordination of and support with any maintenance and updating requirements of the individual's communication methods (e.g., updating and sharing support documentation/information, editing/ updating paper based or electronic systems, setting and reviewing targets/goals). There is a key contact with whom support related advice and guidance can be provided or discussed and they are likely to respond to this and implement strategies.

4 Consistent support. Client has consistent support across all their environments/ settings. Most of the client's everyday communication partners have knowledge of strategies for supporting communication (such as giving time, pausing, using aided language modelling) and recognize the impact of their role as a communication partner. There are many communication partners (in most or all environments) who are aware of and able to support the individual's communication methods. Client is provided with regular opportunities to communicate. There is some coordination of and support with any maintenance and updating requirements of the individual's communication methods (e.g., updating and sharing support documentation/information, editing/ updating paper based or electronic systems, setting and reviewing targets/ goals). There is a key contact with whom support related advice and guidance can be provided or discussed and they are responsive to this and have a plan to implement strategies. They are aware of evidence-based practice.

5 Excellent support. Client has a wide range of supportive communication partners across all their environments/settings. All of the client's everyday communication partners have knowledge of strategies for supporting communication (such as giving time, pausing, using aided language modelling) and recognize the impact of their role as a communication partner. All of the client's everyday communication partners are aware of and able to fully support the individual's communication methods. Client is consistently provided with appropriate opportunities to communicate. There is well coordinated support with any maintenance and updating requirements of the individual's communication methods (e.g., updating and sharing support documentation/ information, editing/updating paper based or electronic systems, setting and reviewing targets/goals). There is a key contact with whom support related advice and guidance can be provided or discussed and they are highly responsive to this and have a plan to implement strategies. They are knowledgeable with regards to evidence-based practice and are proactive in their approach to support.

Acknowledgement: Compiled by the national AAC working party for outcome measures.
Accompanying scale for Therapy Outcome Measure in line with principles detailed in: *Enderby P., John A., Therapy Outcome Measures for Rehabilitation Professionals* 3rd ed. Guildford: J&R Press.

6 Participation in Learning: Child Language Impairment/Phonological Disorder/Dysfluency/ Autistic Spectrum

The Hampshire County Council SEND Speech and Language Therapy Team have developed this scale to provide additional information which reflects how the individual student is able to participate in their learning environment, engage with their learning experience and integrate appropriately in the classroom. Whilst the participation scale in TOM reflects issues beyond the classroom we have found that focusing on classroom integration, and specifically the student's engagement in learning, gives us more detailed information for discussion with teachers and reflecting clear and positive changes as a result of our work.

Participation

0 Unable to engage in any learning or educational role. Not accessing the curriculum.

1 Very limited access to learning for short periods or in some situations.

2 Some participation in class and learning in around 30–40% of lessons.

3 Able to achieve participation in 40–60% of educational activities.

4 Learning for 60–85% of the school day.

5 Achieving learning and educational potential at least 85% of the time and making good progress in all academic areas.

Social integration (in class)

0 No social integration with peers.

1 Limited social integration and socially isolated (in class).

2 Some social integration with peers and able to join in some group activities (in class).

3 Social integration with minimal adult support (in class).

4 Occasional difficulties integrating or fulfilling social role/activity (in class).

5 Achieving learning and educational potential at least 85% of the time and making good progress in all academic areas.

Concentration

1 Highly distracted, disengaged or disruptive.

2 Able to make contributions and demonstrate knowledge occasionally.

3 Able to concentrate with some prompting.

4 Participates in all lessons with occasional disengagement or lapses of concentration or behaviour.

5 Achieving learning and educational potential at least 85% of the time and making good progress in all academic areas.

Progress/Potential

0 No progress being made over a long period.

1 Cannot achieve potential in any situation. Very minimal progress.

2 Making some limited progress in all areas of the curriculum.

3 Making some progress in all areas of the curriculum. Beginning to learn at or around potential but needs some encouragement.

4 May have difficulty in achieving potential in some situations occasionally.

5 Achieving learning and educational potential at least 85% of the time and making good progress in all academic areas.

Acknowledgement: Alison Davies in collaboration with Hampshire County Council SEND Speech and Language Therapy Team and Communication and Language Team.